Dedication

To my Light Family

**For Our Spiritual Evolution in peace,
in love and in connection to Source**

May Great Spirit bless us in mind,
body and heart-soul

Sabina M. DeVita's
Vibrational Cleaning©

"Real Green Essentials: Making Women Healthier"

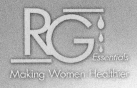

Making Women Healthier

Sabina M. DeVita's

Vibrational Cleaning ©

Real-**G**reen clean...
cancer- and allergy-
proof your home
or office with
Vibrational Cleaning
for vibrancy, wellness,
energy, youthfulness
and more!

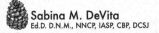

Sabina M. DeVita
Ed.D. D.N.M., NNCP, IASP, CBP, DCSJ

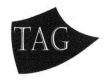

Available From:

Wellness Institute of Living and Learning

7700 Hurontario St., Suite 408

Brampton, ON Canada L6Y 4M3

(905) 451-4475

info@devitawellness.com

info@energywellnessstudies.com

ISBN: 978-1-59930-426-7

Important Notice

The author makes no claims nor is rendering professional advice or service to the individual reader. The information in this book is intended for educational purposes only. It should not replace the recommendations or advice provided by your physician.

Preface

When I became involved with environmental issues in the 1980's, I had no idea how far this path would take me. I was ill with environmental sensitivities, also known as ecological illness or multiple chemical sensitivities (MCS). I experienced brain fog, fatigue, depression, headaches, red burning eyes and malaise. My allergies and chemical sensitivities forced me to change my life path dramatically.

Due to my illness, I turned my attention to natural healing methods and to researching what was then a new phenomenon: environmental health. I discovered how toxic our world had become with environmental toxins, chemical inhalants, pollutants, smog and chemical poisons in our food, water and air. My reactions to the environment were so severe at times that I was not able to drive: Car fumes made me feel drugged, to the point of falling asleep at the wheel. I began to observe how these reactions were affecting my emotions and moods. With this new knowledge, I left my position as a guidance counselor & teacher to pursue a doctoral degree in psychology specializing in **brain allergies**, a rare combination scarcely known or considered for mental health issues—even to this day; **"Brain Allergies"** are rarely considered as a major factor in our mental and emotional well-being.

My university dissertation became the first work of its kind in the field of psychology at the University of Toronto— in fact, it was the first of its kind on **'brain allergies'** and in environmental or ecological sciences. In the years that followed, I became involved with a number of environmental groups: supporting them in their pursuit for cleaner and safer environments, personal care and household products. Our work includes protecting endangered species, conserving wild plant life and literally protecting ourselves.

Over the course of the last 28 years, I have been in private practice utilizing **cutting-edge energy healing practices and energy technologies**. I sourced the finest organic, safe, whole-natured botanicals, herbs and healing products. In the late 1990s, **I discovered the power of organic, therapeutic Grade-A essential oils and the art & science of French medicinal aromatherapy**. These precious and live-food essential oils were introduced into my practices and into all of my natural healing classes.

Over the years, as I taught and learned about the essential oils for body, mind and spirit, I wanted to create a way that the oils could be incorporated into every home. In 2012, I created

Real Green Essentials© as a platform to promote, educate and further the mission of greening every home in shifting consciousness! My Real Green Essentials© environmental initiative is not just to offer a superior cleaning product, but to change the energy aspects within the home— a way to create a Feng Shui shift of the space itself.

"The significant problems we face today cannot be solved at the same level of thinking we were at when we created them."

- Albert Einstein

This book will help you change your life in two major ways:

1) You'll learn how to clean your space with real, plant-based products that are totally toxin-free— ridding your home of dirt, microbes, pests and other invaders.

2) You will raise your home or office frequencies for well-being, happiness and peace—stimulating longevity, harmony and calmness—by using vibrational and eco-green home cleaning methods! In addition, you will learn how to increase your intuitive abilities and more by stimulating your 3rd eye- Pineal gland all while cleaning!

In this book, I will give you what you need to create an eco-friendly, Real Green Clean, vibrationally attuned home—using 100 percent plant-based food for the Whole: body, mind & soul! These products are so natural and safe that you could eat your cleaning supplies!

You will also learn how to cancer-proof your home, to be chemical-free and allergy-free.

This book will show you how to make your home a safe and comfortable **haven**—and by adding an 'e' for energy, you will make your own *'heaven on Earth'*—a sacred space with a higher frequency, thanks to Vibrational Cleaning© methods.

This book presents novel ideas on how to Clean Green and raise the energy in your home at the same time with a combination of pure, genuine essential oils and easy, practical energy or Feng Shui techniques. I've also included a special chapter on **how to decalcify your pineal gland, often called the 3rd eye, to activate your intuition & your spiritual awareness.**

Create your sacred space, attune your energy and discover how good you can feel with Real Green Essentials: Vibrational Cleaning© for a Healthy Home!

"The intuitive mind is a sacred gift and the rational mind is a faithful servant. We have created a society that honors the servant and has forgotten the gift."

~ Albert Einstein

"The power of intuitive understanding will protect you from harm until the end of your days."

~ Lao-Tzu, Ancient Chinese Philosopher

"The mind always points outside for change, The heart always points within. Only by changing within will the outside be different`

~ Peter Ragnar`

Table of Contents

Foreword

I was so intrigued when I saw the title *Vibrational Cleaning* and was anxious to see what was inside. As I began to read, I was amazed at the tremendous research that Dr. DeVita has done. The information was staggering and could be frightening if we didn't have a natural solution. Because of her own toxic illness, she studied intensely to understand why she was ill and how to heal herself.

Her need took her down a path that now benefits thousands of people looking for help. In our chemically toxic world, we have to do everything we can to keep our environment clean, especially our home environment where we have the greatest control. It is imperative that we keep our bodies strong and healthy, but it is critical that we keep our minds protected from the pollutants that cause dizziness, confusion, upset, anger, and even emotional disorientation that can bring about crimes of aggression against humanity.

Dr. DeVita's knowledge of natural modalities, proper supplementation, and the right foods to eat is immense which she openly shares with everyone. The frequency and vibration of aromatic plants in the form of pure essential oils free from synthetic compounds, is one of the easiest ways to protect ourselves.

Vibrational Cleaning is one of the most valuable books anyone can read who is looking for answers and solutions to living in our polluted and toxic world. This book's life-protecting information and recipes will give you knowledge and understanding, that will enable you to create a plan of action that will bring gratitude, fun, and excitement as you see the results of greater health and wellness, and most of all, life-giving freedom.

–**Mary Young**
Executive Vice President
Young Living Company

Introduction:

Greening our homes
*"If you're not riding the wave of change...
you'll find yourself beneath it."*

**This book 'Real Green Essentials-Vibrational Cleaning'
- making women healthier©'** was written in order to help
conscientious consumers truly 'ride the wave of change'. Real
Green Essentials- Vibrational Cleaning© makes it easier and
more pleasant to transition to a greener lifestyle, getting you
out of pain or illness and instead giving you the ability to heal
yourself, wildlife and the planet.

**Adopting a healthy, ecologically friendly way of life is
essential for physical, mental, emotional and spiritual
wellness in order for mass change to occur which will
become more evident as you progress through this book.**

Not only do toxic chemical environments make us sick but they affect the way you feel and the way you think! Our spaces, our environments shape us, influence us in so many detrimental ways but they can also influence us in many beneficial ways once we know how.

The green movement has exploded into popular culture and is quickly developing. It has left most of us, as consumers, unsure of where to begin and unsure as to which products are truly green and safe to use. A study conducted by the Silent Spring Institute showed that there were **a number of green products that are still considered to be toxic.** In particular, sunscreens and fragranced products—including air fresheners, dryer sheets and perfumes—had the largest number of target chemicals and some of the highest concentrations. Fragrances can trigger asthma and some have been shown to mimic estrogen, including making breast cancer cells grow in laboratory studies.

Sabina DeVita's Real Green Essentials Vibrational Cleaning © features products that are simple and pure: all made with organic, therapeutic Grade-A, genuine essential oils from the largest privately owned organic herb farms and the botanical gardens in the world. These same Eco Green essential oils can be used for greening our homes, greening our pets, greening our environment and remarkably to heal and green ourselves on all levels: body-mind-emotion-spirit, all at the same time! They're even kosher certified!

My *Mission* is to educate, liberate, rejuvenate and shift consciousness to bring wellness, abundance, *peace*, joy, harmony and higher awareness to every home in an easy, fun and heart-filled way. As I look back on my life and the paths that I have taken, I realize that this book has become a culmination of many of my experiences helping to fulfill my life purpose. Eco friendly, harmonized environments allow for safe, peace-filled living spaces. This allows for those that create their home as a sanctuary to also experience peace within them. In tandem with Dr. Wayne Dyer's statement below, peace begins at home:

"How do you get world peace? You get world peace through inner peace. If you've got a world full of people who have inner peace, then you have a peaceful world."

The 'wave of change' begins with new learning and new understandings. Congratulations in reading this book as you have made that first or continued step in creating conscious change. The best purchase in improving your life is through education. Education is the key to freedom and health. With this in mind, I created the **Eco-Essentials consultants' program at the Institute of Energy Wellness Studies** to offer workshops as well as this book to help you learn more about the Greening line of eco-friendly, natural and plant-based organic essential oil products. Learn about the role and potency of essential oils and how to incorporate the Eco Green Essentials' way into your life and your home.

Essential oils encapsulate nature's living energy. They are the natural, aromatic volatile liquids found in shrubs, flowers, trees, pine needles, roots, bushes and seeds. The distinctive components in essential oils defend plants against insects, environmental conditions and disease. They are also vital for a plant to grow, live, evolve and adapt to its surroundings.

Essential oils are extracted from aromatic plant sources via steam distillation. They are highly concentrated and far more potent (high quality distilled oils)—in fact, 60 percent to 70 percent more potent—than dry herbs. These natural green essentials were used 6,000 years ago by the Egyptians in all facets of their lives and their benefits have now been re-discovered in our modern world. Therapeutic grade or food-grade organic, medicinal essential oils are truly 100 percent plant-based products.

This book will give you many ideas and methods as a homeowner to get started. I also encourage you to JOIN our green movement and help us shift consciousness by becoming an Eco Green consumer. It's easy to make a difference and very rewarding to help YOU while helping Mother Earth, aquatic life, wildlife, pets and all of humanity! For consultants' workshops, contact the Institute of Energy Wellness Studies found in the appendix.

Enjoy 'Real Green Essentials: Vibrational Cleaning©,' make your home *'heaven on earth'* by introducing 'soul-full' food for your home, your planet and your body!

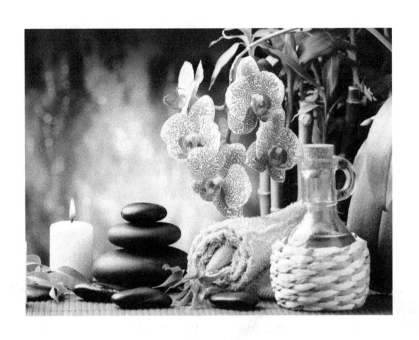

CHAPTER 1:

Our toxic chemical load!

*"We are all part of the environment:
What we do to the environment,
we do to ourselves."*

– Greenpeace

CHAPTER 1:

Who would have thought that staying home could be hazardous to your health? We're now finding that it may even kill you or a family member!

When a participant in one of my classes shared the story of a 3 year old child, who had to be rushed to the hospital after tasting a toxic laundry cleaner, that not only gave him immediate burns but resulted in hours of surgery for a liver transplant at Sick Children's hospital in Toronto, I knew that much more education was needed about toxic home cleaners and personal care items. Many families are unaware of the poisons looming in their homes.

"Toxins in U.S. homes now account for 90 percent of all reported poisonings each year," says Rose Ann Soloway, Administrator of the American Association of Poison Control Centers (AAPCC). On average, U.S. poison control centers handle **one poison exposure every 13 seconds! This is an outrageous statistic.**

Most poisonings involve everyday household items such as medicines, cleaning supplies, cosmetics and personal care items. According to the AAPCC, the most common forms of poison exposure for children under the age of six are cosmetics and personal care products (13.4 percent), cleaning substances (9.8 percent), analgesics (8.2 percent) and foreign bodies (7.4 percent). In 2012, the US poison control centers received reports of 6,271 exposures to highly concentrated packets of laundry detergent by children 5 and younger. 50.7 percent of poison exposures occur in children under the age of six annually.

Even more surprisingly, 92.7 percent of all poison exposures occur in the home—not in industry, as you might expect. The impact of the environmental pollutants over the years has been increasing both in our homes and in our environment. Today's statistics of indoor air pollution are shocking. **Indoor air pollution alone kills one person every 20 seconds! The U.S. Environmental Protection Agency considers indoor air to be one of the four most urgent environmental health risks in North America.**

People spend a large part of their lives indoors: The quality of indoor air is an essential determinant of a healthy life and well-being. In order to make the necessary changes, you must first understand the hazards.

In 2010, the World Health Organization released a report which emphasized that clean air is a basic requirement of life. The report states that every year, indoor air pollution is responsible for the death of 1.6 million people. It claims that

90 percent of chronic illnesses are related to environmental factors. Less than 2 percent of the 80,000 known household chemicals have been tested—and shockingly, many of them contain known neurotoxins.

The average indoor environment contains hazardous chemicals in concentrations 10 to 40 times greater than outdoor air. In tests on blood, urine and breast milk, Environmental Working Group researchers in the U.S. also identified the presence of 455 synthetic chemicals that should not be found in the human body. EWG researchers also found that **the average adult is exposed to 126 chemicals every day just from using personal care products**, including a substance used in anti-freeze and brake fluid that finds its way into moisturisers and shower gels!

One in every 13 women is exposed to a known or a probable human carcinogen every day. In one shocking recent study, researchers at the University of Reading in the UK found that 99 percent of all tissue samples taken from 40 women who had undergone mastectomies for breast cancer contained at least one paraben—and that 60 percent of the samples contained five or more parabens. Parabens are known to have an estrogen-mimicking effect and estrogen is commonly known to play a key role in the development, growth and progression of breast cancer.

The chemical onslaught is staggering

- Since 1965, more than 4 million distinct chemical compounds have been formulated.

- At least 250,000 new formulations are created annually.

- Approximately 3,000 chemicals are added to our foods.

- 700 chemicals have been found in our drinking water.

- 400 chemicals have been identified in human tissues.

- More than 500 chemicals on average can be found in American homes.

- Over 800 neurotoxic chemical compounds have been used in the cosmetic and perfume industries.

Other points to consider:

- ✓ Since the chemical and cosmetic industry is unregulated - chemical manufacturers are not required to list the ingredients on their cleaning products as they're considered, 'trade secrets'.

- ✓ Cleaning products are only required to warn the consumer with labels marked as: Poison, Danger, or Warning!

- ✓ The typical home contains over 63 hazardous products!

CHEMICALS AND YOUR HEALTH

Of the 80,000 Chemicals Being Used Commercially in This Country The EPA Considers 65,000 of Them To be Potentially, if not Definitely, Hazardous to Your Health!

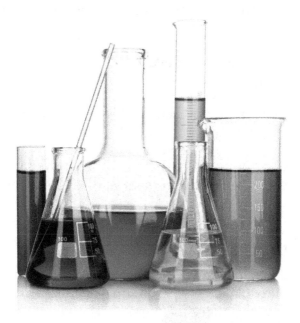

Pat Thomas is the author of '*Cleaning Yourself to Death*', which exposes the chemical-related health risks in the products we use every day. Thomas reports that less than a quarter of the 70,000 to 80,000 chemicals used in toiletries and cleaning products have been subjected to a full safety investigation. Others, officially classed as hazardous waste, are frequently found in products from baby lotion to eye drops and cleaning fluids. In an article for *The Observer*, William Peakin writes:

> *Thomas found high levels of sodium lauryl sulphate, a harsh detergent commonly used as an engine degreaser, in toothpastes, shampoos and cleansers. One of the most dangerous chemicals Thomas found was nitrosamine, a carcinogenic commonly used in baby and body lotions, facial moisturizers and shampoos.*

> *"In the 1970s nitrosamine contamination of bacon and other cured meat became a worldwide public health issue," she said. "A typical portion of bacon will now contain a single microgram of nitrosamine. The amount of nitrosamine that could be absorbed from a single dose of shampoo, on the other hand, is often 100 times that."*

And yet how many people are even aware of this!

Dr. Mercola reveals in a 2013 recent article how air pollution and chemicals found in common household and personal care goods are major sources of exposure that can lead to an accumulation of toxins in the body. A typical American comes in regular contact with some 6,000 chemicals and an untold number of potentially toxic substances on a less frequent basis. Many of them have never been fully tested for safety. In order to protect your health, it's important to take the necessary steps to decrease your chemical exposure, by becoming educated about them. This is certainly one of the major reasons for my authoring this book. Consumers beware.

Dr. Mercola reports on a recent account by *Scientific American* that found chemicals in personal care products such as deodorants, lotions and conditioners, to be detectable in downtown Chicago air samples at "alarming" levels. The chemicals in question were the **cyclic siloxanes** known to be toxic to aquatic life. According to Keri Hornbuckle, an engineering professor at the University of Iowa, 'these airborne compounds are pervasive all around us.' ×°

Michael Dufresne, a leading researcher in environmental cancers, told *CBC Marketplace, that* **"Women who work in the home are at a 54 percent higher risk of developing cancer than career women"**.

All women are exposed to an onslaught of household chemicals and more so for those who are in the home all day long.

Breast cancer

Breast cancer is the most prevalent type of cancer in women and is the leading cause of death among women between the ages of 40-55. The disease's occurrence has risen from one chance in twenty in 1950, to the current rate of one in eight. In the U.S., the rate of breast cancer among white women from 1950 to 1989 increased by 53 percent —over 1 percent annually.

Organochlorine pesticides have been shown to cause breast cancer in rats. Organochlorines are also produced in the manufacture of herbicides, **detergents,** spermicidal foam or lubricants, petrochemicals such as polychlorinated biphenyls (PCBs), PVC plastics and paper.

Environmental pollution

A federal study released in 2012 found more than 100 toxic substances making their way through wastewater treatment plants into the Columbia River.

"In the past people thought of pollution in the river in terms of smokestack industry on the river or dirty pipes," said Jennifer Morace, the U.S. Geological Survey hydrologist who was lead investigator on the study.

"This links it back to what we do in our everyday lives, what goes down the drain and to the wastewater treatment plant, and the fact that they were not designed to remove the new or emerging contaminants."

A total of 112 toxic materials were found—53 percent of those that were tested for—including flame retardants, pharmaceuticals, pesticides, personal care products, mercury and cleaning products.

In a 1990 EPA survey, **every single person tested showed some evidence of petrochemical pollution in their body tissues and fat.**

Some of the chemicals held in the fat cells include styrene (plastics), xylene (solvent in paint and gasoline), benzene (a chemical found in gasoline) and toluene (another carcinogenic solvent).

THE TRICLOSAN THREAT

Triclosan is a toxic product that is causing reproductive and many other types of problems. A common anti-bacterial agent, it is found in a variety of consumer products—everything from antibacterial dish soap to shampoo, toothpaste…even clothing. Products with triclosan are known as "antimicrobials"—substances that inhibit the growth of harmful bacteria, viruses and fungi. Triclosan has been used in consumer products for more than 30 years. It was used relatively rarely through the 1990s, but today is found in nearly 1,000 products.

The Centers for Disease Control and Prevention says that small amounts of the chemical can be absorbed by a person's skin. Although it is not used in any food products, one study found that nearly **<u>75 percent of people</u> tested positive for triclosan in their urine**.

While triclosan is legally considered safe for humans in rinse-off applications like soaps and shampoos, studies show that it is contributing to the surge in life-threatening, antibiotic-resistant super germs and severe hormone disruption in wildlife, cancer and heart disease. It is a known endocrine disruptor, which can cause **thyroid problems and cancer** due to triclosan's structural similarity to **thyroid hormones,** which orchestrate growth and development in wildlife and humans. Triclosan also contaminates the environment, washing down our drains to pollute rivers and lakes. *"When it's found in waterways, for example, male frogs literally sport female parts,"* reports Rodale.com.

Antibacterial soaps are tied to a public health crisis?

Another common complaint is how **triclosan contributes to a surge in mutated, harder-to-kill bacteria or "superbugs".** Recently, Health Canada recommended avoiding antibacterial products because they kill good bacteria that fight bad germs and because of the concerns over antimicrobial resistance. Virulent strains of bacteria are now resistant to triclosan such as *E. coli, Salmonella enterica, Staphylococcus aureus and Mycobacterium tuberculosis*- which are able to fight triclosan with a cellular mechanism. xii

Antibiotic-resistant infections—called MRSA—**street name, 'flesh-eating disease'** now claim more lives each year than the "modern plague" of AIDS and cost the American health care system some $20 billion a year. According to a 2007 study published in the Journal of the American Medical Association, more than 18,600 people died from invasive MRSA infections in the United States in 2005. Those numbers are growing!

And that's just ONE antibiotic-resistant bug. The list of resistant microbes is steadily increasing.

The CDC calls antibiotic resistance **one of the most pressing health issues facing the United States.** Infections caused by bacteria with resistance to at least one antibiotic have been estimated to kill more than 60,000 hospitalized patients each year.

Though triclosan has been measured in house dust, most people are likely to be exposed by applying products that contain triclosan to their skin. One study of nursing mothers found higher levels of triclosan in blood and breast milk of women who used personal care products containing triclosan. It is most commonly used in **hand soaps, cleaning supplies** and **dish detergents**, but also in products that don't claim to be antibacterial. Some toothpastes, kitchen utensils, garbage bags, toys, **computer keyboards, clothing, mattresses, cutting boards** and bedding contain triclosan. Health Canada has also registered 1,200 cosmetics with this ingredient. But the worst offender is **hand sanitizers!**

More environmental concerns

A recent study found that one-third of the bottlenose dolphins tested off South Carolina and almost one-quarter of those tested off Florida carried traces of triclosan in their blood, at concentrations known to disrupt hormones, growth and development in other animals.

Triclosan is one of the most frequently detected chemicals in streams across the U.S., and both triclosan and its neighbor triclocarban are found in high concentrations in sediments and sewage sludge (where they can persist for decades). In the environment, antibacterial compounds could disrupt aquatic ecosystems and pose a potential risk to wildlife. Traces of triclosan have been found in earthworms from agricultural fields and Atlantic dolphins. In the lab, triclosan has been shown to interfere with development of tadpoles into frogs, a process that is dependent on thyroid hormones.

▶ *Triclosan is among the class of chemicals that accumulate to higher and higher concentrations with each step up the food chain. Every creature on earth has these pollutants in its body fat.*

▶ *Once absorbed into the fat cells, **it is nearly impossible to eliminate these compounds.***

Humans are among the animals at the top of the food chain. The health risks are considerable and lethal!

Dr. Joseph Mercola reports another lethal connection with triclosan. Triclosan laden products such as toothpaste, deodorant and antibacterial soap have been linked to heart disease and heart failure.

Researchers at the University of California found that triclosan impairs muscle function and skeletal muscle contractibility. Although the study was done in mice, researchers reported that the effects of the chemical on cardiac function were "dramatic."

Ban triclosan

A recent study of over 200 households found that people using antibacterial products were not actually lowering their risk for contracting viral infections. Triclosan has not been shown to have an added health benefit and the long term effects of chronic low-grade exposure in humans are unknown.

People should not be brushing their teeth and washing their dishes with a cancer-causing chemical. Environmental Defence is currently calling on Health Canada to ban household use of triclosan.

Live safely NOW: some guidelines

- Avoid personal care products labeled "antibacterial" or antimicrobial" and any containing triclosan or triclocarban, such as soaps, gels, cleansers, **toothpaste**.

- Avoid treated "antibacterial" or "antimicrobial" items such as cutting boards, towels, yoga mats, shoes, clothing and bedding- even garbage bags.

- Use natural non-chemical soaps and hot water to clean effectively. Use alcohol-based hand sanitizers like the Eco Green **Thieves Sanitizer©** when you don't have access to running water.

MORE HARMFUL HOUSEHOLD CHEMICALS TO AVOID

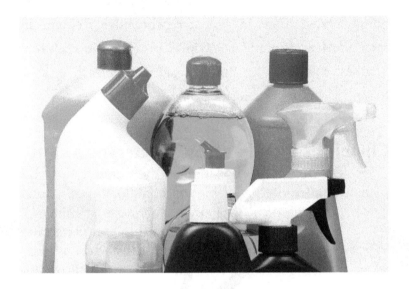

A 2012 Center for Disease Control (CDC) study detected a total of 212 chemicals in the blood and urine samples from a representative sample of 2,400 people nationwide.

Little is known about the human health effects of most of these chemicals. But animal research links exposure to some of them to increased rates of cancer, infertility and stunted organ development.

Below are other chemicals that have been found at high concentrations in the population and that can cause adverse health effects. The chemical industry claims that these chemicals are safe at current exposure levels.

Bleach

Bleach of any kind is considered to be quite toxic by many of the environmental groups. It is now being linked to the rising rates of **breast cancer in women**, **reproductive problems in men** and **learning and behavioral problems in children.** The best solution is to simply avoid using bleach in your home. (See more on chlorine below)

Chemicals found in typical detergents

- **Dioxane (1,4-dioxane)** – The majority of top laundry detergent brands contain this synthetic petrochemical, a known carcinogen. This is a by-product contaminant of the manufacturing process and is not required to be listed on product labels. (See Chapter 3 for more on 1,4-dioxane)

- **DEA (Diethanolamine)** – Found in more than 600 home and personal care products, such as shampoos, conditioners, bubble baths, lotions, cosmetics, soaps, laundry and dishwashing detergents. Suspected of carcinogenic activity (causing or contributing to cancer) or of being potentially dangerous or hazardous to health.

- **Propylene Glycol** – The main ingredient found in *anti-freeze*; also common in shampoos, deodorants, cosmetics, lotions, toothpastes, processed foods, baby wipes, and many more personal care items. Implicated in contact dermatitis, kidney damage and liver abnormalities; can inhibit skin cell growth in human tests and can damage cell membranes causing rashes, dry skin and surface damage.

- **Talc** –The Cancer Prevention Coalition lists Talc as a carcinogen as it is closely related to the potent carcinogen asbestos. Talc particles have been shown to cause tumors in the ovaries and lungs of cancer victims. For the last 30 years, scientists have closely scrutinized talc particles and found dangerous similarities to asbestos. Despite a 1973 ruling about the dangers of talcum, no ruling has ever been made - today, cosmetic grade talc remains non-regulated by the federal government. Talc is used in a wide variety of consumer products ranging from home and garden pesticides to antacids. However, the products most widely used and that pose the most serious health risks are body powders, especially baby powders. The common household hazard posed by talc is inhalation of baby powder by infants. Talc is the principal ingredient in home and garden pesticides and flea and tick powders. Talc is used in smaller quantities in deodorants, chalk, crayons, textiles, soap, insulating materials, paints, asphalt filler paper and in food processing. http://www.preventcancer.com/consumers/cosmetics/talc.htm

- **Alcohol** – Most mouthwash products have higher alcohol content than most alcoholic beverages (beer, wine, etc.). Mouthwash products with alcoholic content greater than 25 percent have been linked to cancers of the mouth, tongue, and throat. Alcohol acts as a solvent inside the mouth, making tissues more vulnerable to carcinogens.

- **Linear Alky Benzene Sulfonates (LAS)** – Synthetic petrochemicals that biodegrade slowly, making them an environmental hazard. Benzene may cause cancer in humans and animals.

- **Nonylphenol Ethoxylate (NPE)** – Petrochemical surfactant banned in the EU and Canada. May cause liver and kidney damage. Biodegradable, but biodegrades into more toxic substances.

- **Petroleum distillates (aka napthas)** – Derived from synthetic crude oil, linked to cancer, lung and mucous membrane damage.

- **Sodium Lauryl Sulfate (SLS)** – Chemical foaming agent known as a surfactant. Studies have linked use of this chemical to a variety of health issues from skin irritation to organ toxicity. Industrial uses include concrete floor cleaners, **engine degreasers** and car wash detergents. Also found in shampoos, liquid soaps, conditioners, cleansers, toothpaste, and children's personal care products. SLS is found in nearly all toothpastes and is absorbed through skin contact and retained for up to five days.

There are 15,965 studies in the PubMed science library relating to the potential risks of SLS. **It's dangerous to your body and to the environment.**

The David Suzuki Foundation notes that, while sodium lauryl sulfate in its pure form is only "moderately" likely to cause organ toxicity, it is highly irritating to your skin and eyes. To solve this, it is often treated with ethylene oxide, resulting in sodium laureth sulfate—a known carcinogen!

According to World Health Organization's International Chemical Safety Card, SLS is a substance that is toxic to aquatic organisms. **The report has strongly advised not to let the chemical enter into the environment. How absurd that this chemical is still being allowed to be used in soaps and shampoos, shower gels etc. and then flushed down the drain into the water table!**

Chlorine

The Dioxin TOXIN: Dioxins are unintended by-products of many chemical and combustion processes which involve chlorine. Dioxin is believed to be **one of the most significant carcinogenic chemicals known to science.**

Dioxin pollution is pervasive in our environment and has quickly moved up the food chain into our food supply. The major source of dioxin in the environment comes from waste-burning incinerators of various sorts, and it is associated with paper mills which use chlorine bleaching in their process. Dioxin is also used with the production of Polyvinyl Chloride (PVC) plastics and with the production of certain chlorinated chemicals (including many pesticides).

Because dioxins accumulate in fatty tissue, **they are found mostly in meat, fish and dairy products. Unfortunately, when people consume these foods, they also consume dioxins.**

The EPA first announced that it would assess the dangers of dioxins in 1985, but did not release a conclusive report for nearly three decades. What important information was it hiding?

According to the Energy Justice Network, the EPA described dioxin as **a serious public health threat—perhaps more dangerous than DDT**—in its 1994 draft report. It reported that dioxin-like chemicals had been found in the general US population and were associated with adverse health effects.

The Center for Health, Environment & Justice released "The American People's Dioxin Report" to help provide more complete information. According to the report, **dioxin exposure causes cancer as well as severe reproductive and developmental problems.** The CHEJ reports that the most striking finding is the impact of dioxin on the growth and development of children—notably its effects on the development of the immune, reproductive, and nervous systems, including cognitive and learning abilities. **For most people, exposure occurs through ingestion of many common foods; unborn children are at the highest risk.** They are exposed to the toxic effects of dioxin during the most sensitive, vulnerable and critical time periods of development in the womb.

Dioxin exposure has also been linked to birth defects, inability to maintain pregnancy, decreased fertility, reduced sperm counts, endometriosis, diabetes, learning disabilities, immune system suppression, lung problems, skin disorders, lowered testosterone levels and much more.

The most toxic compound is 2,3,7,8-tetrachlorodibenzo-p-dioxin or TCDD. TCDD is widely recognized to be carcinogenic to humans. The World Health Organization classifies it as a Group 1 carcinogen, which means that it is known to cause cancer in humans.

How to Evade Dioxin: Avoid chlorinated products like bleached paper towels, disposable diapers, bleached white flour, sugar and tea bags. The more the population demands environmentally friendly, **non-chlorinated products and fewer poisonous chemicals** in manufacturing practices, the less we will be in danger from this toxic dioxin load.

Make a difference: Use eco-green alternatives whenever you can.

Formaldehyde

Formaldehyde is described as **"probably the most dangerous substance on the market"** by Dr. Samuel Epstein, Professor Emeritus at the University of Illinois. It has been given a red flag by health agencies, yet this toxicant is still being used in toiletries, cosmetics and dishwashing products.

Formaldehyde is used in hundreds of materials and products, including furniture, wood products, carpeting, paints, and household cleaning products. California took action in 2007 to limit its use in pressed wood products, and the U.S. Congress passed a law in 2010 to do the same. Unfortunately, the proposed regulations needed to implement the federal law—which Congress mandated be in place by January 1, 2013—are stuck in regulatory review limbo.

"Fragrance", "perfume" or "parfum"

According to the *Journal of the American College of Toxicology*, "fragrance" could be any combination of more than **3,000 different synthetic chemical ingredients**. Chemical fragrances pose a serious health risk and are a significant source of indoor air pollution.

A wide range of mainstream fragrances and perfumes, predominantly based on synthetic ingredients, are used in numerous cosmetics, toiletries, soaps and other household products. They are loaded with toxic and often carcinogenic compounds, including formaldehyde, toluene, phthalates and synthetic musk. Because manufacturers are allowed to guard their special blend of fragrance as a trade secret, **none of these 3,000+ chemicals EVER get listed on the label.**

The first synthetic perfume was created in the 2oth century by Coco Chanel. Chanel no. 5 relied heavily on synthetic aldehydes—a toxic chemical which belongs to the same group of toxic chemicals as the carcinogenic formaldehyde and hangover-causing acetaldehyde.

The government agencies that oversee product safety do not systematically review the safety of fragrances. Currently, **the fragrance industry is virtually unregulated.** Its recklessness is abetted and compounded by FDA's complicity. The FDA has refused to require the industry to disclose ingredients due to trade secrecy considerations, and still takes the position that "consumers are not adversely affected, and should not be deprived of the enjoyment" of these products.

The essential oil industry grows and harvests their oils naturally, but sells 98 percent of their products to the perfume and fragrance industry and only 2 percent to the health industry. What a shame that nature's pure, healing perfumes are being polluted with toxins before we are able to reap their benefit!

So-Called "Green" Cleaners

In 2013, the Environmental Working Group released a ground-breaking initiative to uncover the truth about toxic chemicals in common household products. The "Hall of Shame" has unearthed compelling evidence about **hundreds of cleaners that are hyped as "green" or "natural," but that can inflict serious harm on unwary users.** Many of these toxic products present severe risks to children, who may ingest them or breathe their fumes!

For example, EWG points out how many cleaners are labeled "safe," "non-toxic" and "green" and can contain hazardous ingredients. They call this practice **"greenwashing".**

One cleaner that EWG exposes is the Simple Green Concentrated All-Purpose Cleaner, which contains:

- 2-butoxyethanol, a solvent absorbed through the skin that damages red blood cells and irritates eyes

- a secret blend of alcohol ethoxylate surfactants. Some members of this chemical family are banned in the European Union.

EWG comments that the company's website gives instructions for the user to dilute the product significantly for even the heaviest cleaning tasks. Yet it comes in a spray bottle, which implies that it should be sprayed full-strength. Such use, they say, 'would result in higher exposures'.

HORMONE DISRUPTORS AND POISONOUS PLASTICS

Nicholas Kristof, (May, 2012) columnist for *The New York Times*, writes that chemicals—particularly endocrine disrupters—are feminizing male animals in the wild. Male frogs are showing up with female organs, and some male fish actually produce eggs. In a Florida lake contaminated by these chemicals, male alligators have tiny penises. **Last year, eight medical organizations representing genetics, gynecology, urology and other fields made a joint call in Science magazine for tighter regulation of endocrine disruptors.**

<u>Endocrine disruptors</u> are everywhere and are wreaking havoc with the endocrine system that governs hormones. This can cause such conditions as breast cancer, infertility, low sperm counts, genital deformities, early menstruation and even male breast development, along with diabetes and obesity.

They're found in canned foods, cosmetics, plastics, household cleaners, personal care products and food packaging. Worrying new research on the long-term effects of these chemicals is constantly being published. One study found that pregnant women who have higher levels of a common endocrine disruptor, PFOA (Perfluorooctanoic acid, a synthetic chemical that does not occur naturally in the environment), are *three times as likely* to have daughters who grow up to be overweight. Yet PFOA is unavoidable. It is in everything from microwave popcorn bags to carpet-cleaning solutions, non-stick surfaces on cookware and waterproof, breathable membranes for clothing and some paints. Because of its common use, PFOA is found in virtually everyone's blood.

Kristof points out that the incidence of **hypospadias,** a congenital malformation of the penis, has doubled amongst little boys. He writes about the expanding evidence that hypospadias and other birth defects in people and wildlife may be linked to the daily bombardment of endocrine disruptors in household goods, pesticides and other man-made products.

Phlathates

Phthalates are a hormone-disrupting chemical found in personal care products and plastics. These industrial chemicals make plastics flexible and resilient. They show up in numerous everyday products, from car parts to personal care products.

They end up in the body when we swallow and inhale them, and less frequently, when our skin comes into contact with certain products. The health impacts of phthalates haven't yet been measured in humans, but they cause **reproductive and liver problems** in lab rats.

Not only have these chemicals been linked to cancer, but Swedish researchers have presented evidence that **phthalates may double the risk for type 2 diabetes in adults.**

More Estrogen Mimickers Make Males more Feminine!

Phthalates are known reproductive toxins or endocrine disrupters classified as *__xenoestrogens__* (synthetic estrogen hormone mimickers) that make males and females more feminine. More research is linking this chemical to the rising incidence of hormone-related medical conditions such as polycystic ovarian syndrome, infertility and breast cancer in women—and decreased sperm count in men.

The European Commission proposed a ban on the use of phthalates back in 2002, after it was found to be causing infertility in men and genital abnormalities. Cases of *testicular cancer* in young men have risen *tenfold i*n the past century. Phthalates have been shown to damage developing testes in males and places unborn baby boys at highest risk.

In the 1990s, declining semen quality was reported from Belgium, Denmark, France, and Great Britain. The incidence of testicular cancer has also increased during the same time.

Similar reproductive problems occur in many wildlife species, attributable to environmental *xenoestrogens.* Reproductive failure in animals and humans has reached unprecedented levels.

Men are increasingly acquiring female blood characteristics and developing male breasts—a common condition called **gynecomastia.** In many animal studies around the world, scientists are publishing similar findings: emasculated males, male breast growth, decreasing sperm counts, low testosterone and high levels of estrogens in both sexes due to concentrated xenoestrogens. It's not a surprise that **the majority of Americans tested by the Centers for Disease Control and Prevention showed metabolites of multiple phthalates in their urine at any given time.**

With 1 billion pounds of phthalate being produced per year worldwide—to be used in products from plastic shower curtains and plastic water bottles to **shampoo** and **detergents**—it has become impossible to avoid these chemicals completely. The answer lies in consumer awareness and using our pocket book to support non-phthalated as well as non-chemical products. We can **stop buying these toxic household detergents, perfumes, deodorants, air fresheners and shampoos, and opt for greener, cleaner ones.**

Of all the chemicals that contain estrogen, plastics may be the worst because they're everywhere. From plastic bags and

Have you used any of these products recently?

- Detergents
- Shampoo
- Deodorants
- Perfumes
- Hairspray
- Garden hose
- Vinyl flooring
- Moisturizers
- Inflatable toys
- Pesticides
- Fertilizers
- Any plastics

Then you have exposed yourself to phthalates!

Get rid of your plastics and anything that is made with phthalates.

water bottles to the packaging your food comes in, **plastic is impossible to get rid of.**

"Musk"

Synthetic musk—a popular perfume fixative used to stabilize the composition of a perfume or fragrance—is also a dangerous compound, another **xenoestrogen** and a hormone imposter. It was traditionally obtained from the male musk deer, until the demand for musk endangered the deer population. Today, perfume companies use synthetic musk and its compounds. Synthetic musk compounds are **extremely toxic,** causing genetic damage in animal experiments as well as being linked to reproductive and fertility problems, testicular cancer in men, and breast and uterine cancer in women. They have been found in human fat and breast milk, with recent studies showing 5X greater concentrations in breast milk samples compared to studies conducted ten years previously. They are ecologically harmful due to their high dermal permeability in animals and aquatic wildlife.

Organochlorines

Organochlorines are produced in the manufacture of herbicides, detergents (including those present in the production of spermicidal foam or lubricants), petrochemicals such as polychlorinated biphenyls (PCBs), PVC plastics and paper.

Organochlorines are now everywhere. According to Greenpeace, thirteen tons of chlorine are produced in North America every year. One percent is used to chlorinate drinking water, while the rest *(99 percent) is used in the production of plastics, to bleach paper products and for many other* industrial and agricultural uses.

Recent scientific research has clearly demonstrated an association between organochlorines and breast cancer. **In other words, organochlorines mimic estrogen.**

The chemical takes up a receptor site, and can prevent a natural hormone from binding, blocking its normal function. Organochlorines can move into the nucleus of a receptor cell and disrupt the cell's growth and division.

Xenoestrogens like this one are known to *exaggerate the carcinogenic effects of radiation* and may increase the breast cancer risk among women who were subjected to prenatal exposure to these substances.

Bisphenol-A

Coupled with phthalates is another toxic compound, bisphenol-A (BPA). This chemical is commonly used in plastics such as food containers, plastic dinnerware and plastic water bottles, toys, eyeglass lenses, auto parts, CDs and many more. Exposure to BPA is thought to primarily happen when we eat foods that have come into contact with the chemical. It is highly toxic to some animals, interfering with brain and reproductive organ development. Studies in humans are murky, but have found a variety of possible health effects, including a possible association between BPA and heart disease.

HEALTH CANADA'S FINDINGS:

2009-2011 study shows that Most Canadians show BPA in their urine: 95% of Canadians aged three to 79!

In 2007, 38 of the world's leading scientific experts on BPA warned policymakers of potential adverse health effects of exposure to the widespread plastic. The report concluded that:

"BPA alters 'epigenetic programming' of genes in experimental animals and wildlife that results in persistent effects that are expressed later in life. Specifically, prenatal and/or neonatal exposure to low doses of BPA results in organizational changes in the prostate, breast, testis, mammary glands, body size, brain structure and chemistry, and behavior of laboratory animals."

CBC news recently reported the 2009-2011 Health Canada study that was released in April 2013 based on 6,400 Canadians, (http://www.cbc.ca/news/health/story/2013/04/17/health-canada-bpa-lead-urine.html) on environmental chemicals. The report suggests that most Canadians have the chemical bisphenol A in their urine and all have traces of lead in their blood. The study shows BPA was detected in the urine of **95 per cent of Canadians aged three to 79.** Children aged three to five and six to 11 had the highest average concentration of BPA, while adults 60 to 79 had the lowest average level. Most significant about the study was the chemical exposures found amongst the most vulnerable group – our children.

BECOME A CONSCIOUS AND CHANGE AGENT CONSUMER

We are all exposed to these toxic compounds throughout our lifetime, without ever knowing it. Many people have been duped into believing that if it's sold in a store than it must be safe—after all, our governments would regulate it if it wasn't! Of course this is the furthest from the truth: **The chemical industry works non-stop to produce new synthetic chemicals. In fact, over 100,000 chemicals are in use in different areas of our lives today, with 5 percent or less having been thoroughly tested for their safety on human health or the environment.**

If it wasn't for my own chemical sensitivities awakening me to these dangers, I too would have been blinded as to the true causes of many illnesses and conditions. **It should not take a health crisis to make us aware of the toxic soup we're living in! Unfortunately, it is often the case.**

With the modern advancements of the information age—particularly the Internet—we now have a faster vehicle to alert our neighbors to a better, safer and cleaner way. **It is our moral and conscientious responsibility to share this awareness and save ourselves, our children and the planet.** The material presented thus far certainly shows a most grim and toxic world. By joining together to diminish the planet's toxic burden and to stop the destruction of plant, wildlife and human lives will improve our chances of a happy, vibrant, healthy life. The power of unity will ride the wave of change.

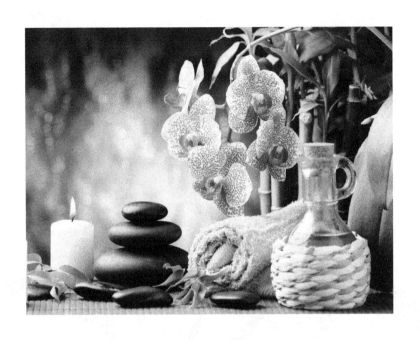

CHAPTER 2:

Why Essential Oils?

"Aromatic plants have been the object of respect and veneration among the majority of civilizations of the past."

- Dr. Daniel Pénoël

CHAPTER 2:

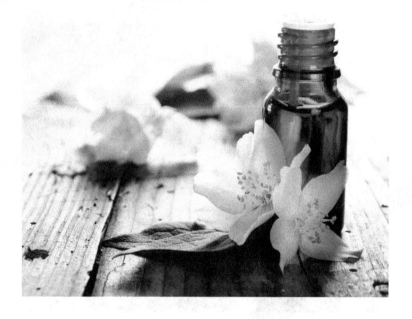

As the number of virulent microbes continues to increase in our communities along with the drug- resistant superbugs due to the overwhelming toxic chemical overload, researchers are paying attention more than ever to the amazing natural cures of essential oils. Modern science has rediscovered the healing, disinfecting and antiseptic properties of essential oils. Over 200 types of essential oils are distilled worldwide today, with several thousand chemical constituents and aromatic molecules identified and registered.

Only 1 percent of essential oils on the world market are used for therapeutic purposes, whereas the rest of the oils grown and distilled are produced for the fragrance and perfume chemical industry. Essential oils have a phenomenal capacity to aid in various ways: anti-bacterial, anti-fungal, anti-viral, anti-parasitic, antiseptic and disinfectant as well as restoring and regenerating skin cells. **When used in cleaning agents, essential oils disinfect and cleanse while healing the body, mind and emotions through inhalation.** They destroy infectious agents in the environment, in food and on skin.

They help to relieve stress and tension; when diffused or used as an air freshener, they help to calm and relax you. They stimulate skin cells into reproducing at a quicker rate, thus reducing the time lag between new skin growth and elimination of old cells and helping to reverse the process of aging. Furthermore, essential oils are fast acting: quickly absorbed by inhalation (within milliseconds) or directly through the skin.

THE POWER OF CONCENTRATION

Because of the tiny molecular structure of the components of an essential oil, they are extremely concentrated. One drop contains approximately 40 million-trillion molecules[i]. Numerically, that is a 4 with 19 zeroes after it:

$$40,000,000,000,000,000,000$$

We have 100 trillion cells in our bodies, and that's a lot. But **one drop of essential oil contains enough molecules to cover every cell in our bodies with 40,000 molecules.**

Considering that it only takes one molecule of the right kind to open a receptor site and communicate with the DNA to alter cellular function, you can see why even inhaling a small amount of oil vapor can have profound effects on the body, brain and emotions.

WHAT ARE ESSENTIAL OILS?

Simply stated, essential oils are distilled from shrubs, flowers, roots, trees, pine needles, bushes and seeds as a subtle, aromatic, volatile liquid. **They are the lifeblood or the life-force of the plant, containing the regenerating and oxygenating immune defense properties of the plants.** They are sometimes referred to as the heart, soul or spirit of aromatic plants. They are the source of all fragrance in plant life. Essential oils have distinctive components so as to defend plants against insects, environmental conditions and disease. All organic and therapeutic oils are powerful and safe, without side effects.

Essential oils are volatile, which means they vaporize quickly into the air. During vaporization, we are able to detect the scent of aromatic plants.

The term 'essential' is derived from 'quintessence' which means "an extract of a substance containing its principle in its most concentrated forms". The word 'essential' was used for essential oils because they were considered to be the very essence, spirit or life of the plant.

Essential oils are highly concentrated: at least 70 times more potent than what is originally found in plant form. It's the steam distillation or cold pressed extraction that makes them highly concentrated and far more potent than dry herbs. **It takes 4,000 to 5,000 pounds of rose petals (14 acres or rose plants) to make 1 pound of rose oil.**

Essential oils' chemical makeup is complex and their benefits are vast—which makes them much more than something that simply smells good. In recent years, research has uncovered essential oils' added benefit as an antiseptic, antibacterial, antifungal, antiviral with the ability to dissolve toxic chemical compounds and more.

Due to their potency, it is best to keep essential oils out of the eyes, ears and nose. Only therapeutic-grade oils can be applied neat onto the skin. For sensitive skin, dilute with vegetable oil, not water. Follow all label directions for a satisfactory application.

HISTORY OF ESSENTIAL OILS

Essential oils are considered to be mankind's first medicine, dating back to 4500 BC. Ancient Egyptians were the first to discover the power of fragrances and data records show that oils and aromatics were used for treating illness: for performing rituals and religious ceremonies in temples and pyramids. Interestingly, three oils that are still commonly used today—Cedarwood, Myrrh, and Frankincense—were used in the ancient Egyptian embalming process. According to the translation of ancient Egyptian hieroglyphics and Chinese manuscripts, priests and physicians were using essential oils thousands of years before Christ. In temples throughout the ancient Middle East, incense played an important role in religious ritual.

Ancient Egyptian papyrus found in the temple of Edfu, contained formulations to make medicines and perfumes used by the alchemists and high priests. The Egyptians were considered as experts in cosmetology and in their preparations of ointments.

When King Tutankhamen's tomb was opened in 1922, some 50 alabaster jars to hold 350 liters of oil were discovered. Upon testing of the essential oils, they were found, remarkably, to be just as bio-active as they are today.

The Greeks between 500 and 400 B.C were perhaps the first to expand the use of essential oils by successfully applying aromatics to psychological conditions such as anxiety, depression and hysteria as well as to beauty and romance. The Roman emperors were famous for their extravagance. They were excessive users of perfumes and aromatic oils. They had saffron sprayed from fountains and used as a strewing herb.

The emperor Nero (1st century, A.D.) was in a class by himself, though. Flowers rained down from the ceiling in his state dining room and silver pipes hidden in the walls sprayed perfumes upon the guests.

Hippocrates (410 B.C.) may have been the first high profile advocate of aromatic therapy. He was known to recommend that:

"The way to health is to have an aromatic bath and a scented massage every day."

There are over 188 references to aromatics, incense and ointments throughout the Bible; the word 'oil' is mentioned 191 times; and some of these oils, such as, frankincense, myrrh, rosemary, hyssop and spikenard, were used for anointing and healing of the sick. Biblical prophets recognized the use of essential oils as a protection for their bodies against the ravages of disease. Richly scented anointing oil consecrated Aaron and his descendants as priests.

Balm of Gilead from Israel, cinnamon from India and frankincense, myrrh from the Arabian coast were carried by caravans of up to 300 camels along a trade route that came to be known as the Frankincense Trail. The heavy-laden beasts left a packed trail in the sand. It is still visible to satellites thousands of years later. These caravan trails became the means by which the lost city of Ubar was located.

Aromatics reigned over the ancient world. Fragrance-laden wax cones were worn atop the heads of wealthy Egyptian women, while the herbal concoctions of the great Greek physician Hippocrates healed the sick. The Three Wise Men brought oils of frankincense and myrrh to the Christ Child. *"The Lord hath created medicines out of the earth; and he that is wise will not abhor them"* (Ecclesiasticus 38:4)

Throughout world history, the use of fragrant oils and spices played an important as well as a prominent role in everyday life. Essential oils and other aromatics were used in religious rituals to treat various illnesses and for other physical and spiritual needs. One of the Dead Sea Scrolls on display in Israel at the shrine of the Book Museum contains an important yet intriguing phrase: **"and he will know his children by their scent".**

The Re-Discovery of Essential Oils

The reintroduction of essential oils into modern medicine began during the late 19th and early 20th centuries, thanks to the re-discovery of their therapeutic benefits by Dr. René-Maurice Gattefossé. In 1910 Rene – Maurice Gattefossé M.D. a famous French chemist, scholar and perfumer had inherited the perfumery business from his family. Due to an experiment that he was conducting, he severely burned his hand: he immediately plunged his hand into the nearest tub of liquid which just happened to be lavender essential oil. He was later amazed at how quickly his burn had healed with very little scarring. As a result of his experience, Gattefossé began his fascination with essential oils. He was inspired to experiment with the oils during the First World War on soldiers in the military hospitals. He primarily used lavender, thyme, lemon and clove essential oils for their antiseptic properties and later shared his ground-breaking research with Dr. Jean Valnet, a Paris medical doctor. Dr. Jean Valnet was also a doctor of Psychiatry, Microbiology, and a Physician of the Military who continued essential oil research into World War II. Similarly, Dr. Valnet discovered the healing powers of essential oils to surpass the antibiotic drugs in use at the time.

Dr. Jean Valnet pioneered the **medicinal uses** of essential oils and wrote the "Practice of Aromatherapy" for doctors and also for the general public. His book details his scientific work of 10 years of laboratory experimentation on essential oils. Dr. Jean Valnet stated that the intelligent use of essential oils gives results that no modern therapeutic can obtain. He also warned that essential oils used in aromatherapy must be of *"irreproachable quality, perfectly pure and natural."*

He also affirms in his book that: "Essential oils are especially valuable as antiseptics because their aggression toward microbial germs is matched by their total harmlessness to tissue…(more over) infectious microbes do not appear to become accustomed to the essential oils as they do to many forms of treatment using antibiotics." Clinical research, for example, has now found that frankincense oil contains very high immuno-stimulating properties. Science is currently re-discovering healing substances that were used in ancient times.

"In recent years, both doctors and the public have re-discovered the medical value of essential plant oils, but the idea of using their properties to maintain or regain health goes back to antiquity. The Romans gained their knowledge of essential oils from the Greeks, who in turn, had received it from the Egyptians." – Dr. Jean Valnet, M.D. 1

Today we see essential oils being used for aromatherapy, massage therapy, emotional health, personal care, nutritional supplements, household solutions and much more. They are also used spiritually to balance mood, lift spirits and dispel negative emotions.

POWER OF SMELL: THE NOSE KNOWS!

"Smells are one of the quickest ways to change mood and emotion and can induce memories."

– Dr. Alan R. Hirsch

It is well known that **our most powerful and direct connection to the subconscious is our sense of smell.** There are 800 million nerve endings for processing and detecting odors, instantly sending a myriad of messages to the brain. Our sense of smell is estimated to be 10,000 times more acute than our other senses with sensitivity to some 10,000 chemical compounds. Scents travel more quickly to the brain than do stimuli from sight or sound. The odors induce parts of the brain to stimulate the release of hormones and neuro-chemicals which alters body physiology and therefore human behavior.

Scientists have learned that **oil fragrances may be one of the most effective tools to achieve desired physiological or psychological effects.**

How smell works in the body

When a fragrance is inhaled, the odor molecules travel up the nose where there are countless anatomic and physiologic interconnections through the olfactory bulb, stria and nuclei to the olfactory tubercle, travelling to numerous other limbic-system structures including the amygdala. The olfactory bulb transmits these odor impulses to the gustatory center (where emotional memories are stored), and other parts of the brain that control **heart rate, blood pressure, breathing, memory, stress levels and hormone balance.**

Smell is the only sensory system whose stimuli are processed throughout the limbic portion of the brain before being processed by the thalamus. The thalamus is the relay station to and from the cerebral cortex, like a switchboard which decodes stimuli and sends it to the brain. In other words, **your response to smell is going to be emotional before it can be rational.**

Brain chemistry gets involved in the form of neurotransmitters, chemicals in the brain that allow the nerve impulses from the olfactory bulb to move from neuron to neuron and on through the limbic system. Neurotransmitters serve many functions, including **the regulation of mood and emotional well-being.** Most of the brain's neurotransmitters are located in the olfactory bulb, providing further evidence of the link between human emotions and our sense of smell.

Neurology of Smell: Dr. Alan Hirsch

Dr. Alan R. Hirsch is a neurologist and psychiatrist specializing in the treatment of smell and taste. He has studied the impact of smell on the brain for over 20 years and has written a number of books (and more than 180 articles) on the psychological power of smell, taste and how these senses affect human behavior. Among his many accomplishments, Dr. Hirsch is Neurological Director of the Smell & Taste Treatment and Research Foundation in Chicago, IL.

Hirsch teaches that physiologically, **odors are processed directly to the limbic system**—our emotional switchboard—

which consists of the pineal, pituitary, hypothalamus and amygdala. All of our other senses (touch, taste, hearing, and sight) bypass the limbic system, first being routed through to the thalamus, passing stimuli onto the cerebral cortex, our conscious thought center.

That is to say: **Unlike with our other senses, we react first to smells and think later.**

According to Hirsch, "The limbic lobe is the part of the brain where we store our emotional memories; anxiety, depression, joy, pleasure, anger, and so forth. This is why our sense of smell is such a powerful trigger for nostalgic reverie, based on nothing more than a whiff of an odor on the air."

Dr. Hirsch points out that **odors impact all of us whether we like it or not**. The understanding that odors evoke more powerful reactions than the other senses do is not particularly new. It is well known that the aroma of freshly baked goods conjures up warm childhood memories.

Because human reaction to odors can be so sudden, powerful and irrational, Dr. Hirsch suggests that people can perform a type of self-analysis by taking note of their reactions to particular odoriferous stimuli. Smells influence us in a preconscious way and create impressions— especially in relationships to others. "We are as we smell" he says—and **so if someone smells good, people will tend to think the person is good. Similarly, if someone smells bad, others will not likely react favorably.**

On days when bad smells from air pollution are present, Hirsch notes, there is an increase in motor vehicle accidents due to people driving more aggressively. Behavioral problems amongst school children increase with bad environmental smells. Accordingly, Hirsch states: "We know that bad odors tend to promote aggression and impair learning ability."

Obviously, the type of smells used in your home or office will impact you and more so in a negative way, if they are synthetic in any way.

More research on aroma and the brain

A study at the University of Cincinnati showed that the fragrances of peppermint and lily of the valley **increased subjects' performance accuracy by 15 to 25 percent.**

Another study, conducted over the course of five years at Yale University, found that within a minute of smelling the aroma of spiced apples, subjects produced slower brain waves associated with increased relaxation.

According to a study published in *Psychogeriatrics*, **aromatherapy with lemon essential oil led to a significant improvement in certain measures of cognitive function among Alzheimer's patients.**

Several other studies are suggesting that lemon essential oil may help reduce anxiety and stress. A 2004 study published in *Brain Research* determined that exposure to the odor of lemon essential oil helped reduce levels of corticosterone (a type of stress hormone) in rats. It was also found that lemon essential oil induced chemical changes in the neuronal circuits, showing anxiety-reducing and pain-relieving properties.

Another study, published in *The International Journal of Neuroscience*, proposed that **aromatherapy may be an effective way to ease the anxiety associated with Alzheimer's disease.** The women in the study, who received 20-minute hand massages with rosemary, lavender, lemon, orange and chamomile three times a week showed reduced anxiety and improved self-esteem.

Essential oil aromatherapy:

- Awakens the spirit
- Quiets the mind
- Soothes the emotions
- Supports a detox program
- Rejuvenates the skin and renews the cells
- Supports normalization of the body systems

What does all this mean for you as a homeowner? When you use essential oils added to your cleaning solutions (as described in Chapter 7), **the aroma will diffuse into the air and you will experience the psychological benefits of aromatherapy.** Essential Oils support many healing and uplifting properties (like anti-depressants) when diffused into the air. They can support various health conditions assisting with lowering blood pressure and reducing muscle aches and pains which may be the causes of your stress and anxiety. Using essential oils helps to promote health, healing, physical energy and purification. For you the homeowner, cleaning will now take on a new experience and significance.

OTHER WORLDWIDE RESEARCH

In terms of antiseptics and disinfectants, essential oils have been well researched and tested in their efficacy for a variety of illnesses. Essential oils are represented in almost 10,000 medical studies that can be found on the largest medical library in the world; the U.S. National Library of Medicine (www.pubmed.gov). For example, in a 2010 study at the University of Delaware, *Salmonella enterica* was washed away successfully on grape tomatoes with thyme oil, thymol and carvacrol instead of a chlorine –based washing solution. xii

More advantages to using essential oils in your home: a unique effective, novel way for real green cleaning

1) The aromas help to reduce the bacteria, fungus, mold and viruses in the air. A number of hospitals in the U.S. have introduced Young Living essential oils to fight MRSA – bacterial infections epidemic amongst other issues and

therapies. (See Chapter 3 for more detail)

2) Inhaling the aromas aids in cleansing the pituitary and pineal glands and helps to activate their function, as well as helping to maintain youthfulness. The Pineal gland is an anti-aging gland. This can be called anti-aging cleaning! (Chapter 5)

3) Most of these same essential oils can be used in your smoothies, juices, salad dressings and food preparations. Essential oil is truly a superfood/ raw food/live food. You can also use them for food preservation. (Chapter 7)

4) Due to the oils having the highest frequencies than any other herb or foods, dispensing them in your home/office regularly will also increase the frequency in your home or office. In other words, this becomes another way to maintain a higher vibration in your home. Higher vibrations allow for better health, calmness and happiness. (Chapter 4)

5) The same oils used for cleaning—e.g. Lavender, which can be used as an antiseptic in cleaning or for freshening your linens—can also be used to ward off insects as an insect repellent or treat insect bites. Lavender and many other oils are also effective treatment for scrapes, cuts, burns, headaches and many other health conditions. (Chapter 3, Chapter 7, Chapter 9)

6) The quickest way to emotional balancing and relaxation is through the olfactory system. Relax the body, relieve tension and clear the mind—

all at the same time that you are cleaning, laundering, dusting or washing the dishes.

7) Reduce stress and anxiety feelings at the same time by inhaling essential oils (like Idaho Balsam Fir) which help to reduce cortisol, the stress hormone, also referred to as the death hormone. Most people today are chronically stressed. Just by spritzing the furniture or wiping the counter top you can help reduce your cortisol.

8) Atmospheric oxygen is increased with essential oils, meaning that the oils increase oxygen availability, produce negative ions and release natural ozone.

9) Help to neutralize seasonal allergies. Lavender is known to support anti-histamine actions as well.

10) Some essential oils also aid in sun protection. Spritz your skin as you spritz the counter top, especially with Lavender, Melaleuca, Helichrysum and/or Lemongrass, adding sesame or coconut oil to protect and soften your skin.

11) Balance your home with essential oils and balance your hormones at the same time! Certain essential oils help to support hormonal balance.Help with weight management by the selective use of the essential oil.

12) Improve concentration, alertness and mental clarity.

13) Stimulate neurotransmitters.

14) Improve digestive function.

15) Speed recovery: Inhalation alone speeds healing recovery by **70 percent!**

16) Improve your immune system: essential oils improve the secretion of IgA antibodies and increases immunity by **32 percent**.

17) Some essential oils high in sesquiterpenes (as found by Vienna and Berlin University researchers) such as Cedarwood and Frankincense can increase the levels of oxygen in the brain by up to **28 percent!**

All of the above virtues can be experienced by merely imbuing your environment with Mother Nature's scents— by the simple inhalation of wafts of fragrance in the air. This can only be achieved by using truly, clean, eco-green, therapeutic grade standard essential oils.

How to Earth/Ground yourself with essential oils

Grounding or Earthing is a new-yet-very old concept for re-establishing balance in our nervous systems. More so today, we are so un-grounded by the synthetic, plastic world we live in, the massive chemical insults we are subjected to and by the electromagnetic pollution that we all are exposed to all day long—that **we have become disconnected from the Earth.**

The book, '*Earthing: The Most Important Health Discovery Ever?*' outlines the importance of connecting to Mother Earth. It points out that **the disconnect with our Earth creates abnormal physiology and contributes to inflammation, pain, fatigue, stress and poor sleep.**

By reconnecting to the Earth, like we do when we are out walking barefoot along the water's edge at the beach or on a stretch of dew-moistened grass, many of these symptoms are rapidly relieved and even eliminated; recovery from surgery, injury and athletic overexertion is accelerated. The authors suggest going barefoot outside for a half-hour and seeing what a difference it makes on your pain or stress level.

Sit, stand, or walk on grass, sand, dirt, or even concrete to receive the Earth's benefits. If you are not able to do that during the winter months or if you live in a high-rise, then you can either stand on concrete floors in your basement to stay connected, for example, or use other simple and inexpensive ways to stay connected. **I suggest that we invite Mother Earth into our homes all the time by utilizing essential oils. Let the fragrance of the conifer trees, the flowery plants or herbs bless your surroundings while grounding you, especially in using the grounding oils.** You can achieve so many healing benefits in a very simple way.

Let Earth Day be every day in your home: get grounded by diffusing your favorite oil for relaxing, for concentration or for harmony. **Utilize essential oils as outlined in this book:**

for your household cleaning and to capture the best of the plant kingdom within you and your home.

Grounding tip: Apply the oils of **Valor***, **Grounding***, **Idaho Balsam Fir, Spruce, Fir, or Blue Spruce** directly onto your feet. It's a great way to rebalance your nervous system.

(* Proprietary blends by Young Living Essential Oil company)

QUALITY OF ESSENTIAL OILS - WORD OF CAUTION

As was mentioned earlier in this chapter, only 1 percent of essential oils on the world market are used for therapeutic purposes, whereas the rest of the oils grown and distilled are produced for the fragrance and perfume chemical industry. This means that there are very few companies in the world that produce essential oils that are unadulterated, chemical free, safe and pure that are also edible as a dietary food as well as topically effective. I specifically chose the Young Living company to write about after researching the many companies that espouse their purity today and are not. Buyers beware! There are many who mimic in words.

Remember Dr. Valnet warned that essential oils used in aromatherapy must be of *"irreproachable quality, perfectly pure and natural"*. *It would make no 'sense' for me to recommend the use of 'scents' to you for the benefits outlined previously, by using inferior, adulterated (often during distillation) essential oils. Why would you want to inhale a potential chemical toxin that was used in the distilling process of the oil?*

Many of the essential oils produced in the world market today are processed with chemical solvents rendering them unsafe for therapeutic purposes. For example, much of the lavender oil that is sold in the American market is a hybrid called lavendin which is grown and distilled in China, Russia, France and Tasmania. To improve the fragrance it is imported into France where it is cut with synthetic linalyl acetate. Other solvents (propylene glycol, DEP or DOP-phthalates) are added to increase the volume and sold in the United States as lavender oil.

Another example is Frankincense that is commonly adulterated to make the essential oil less expensive. The Frankincense oil resin is costly, sold on the world market between $30,000. and $35,000. per ton. It takes a great deal of time to steam distill this essential oil (12 hours or more) thus making the oil quite expensive. It sells inexpensively on the world market as it is cheaply distilled with alcohol or other solvents (like diethyl phthalate, DEP) leaving the essential oil laden with toxic chemicals. (xii)

For this reason and many others mentioned in this section, there are very few companies in the world (a few small companies) that adhere to the rigor in the growing practices and distillation process to produce therapeutic high quality essential oils as does Young Living who grows and distills on their own organic, solvent-free, chemical free, environmentally sustainable farms!

Here is a guideline to help you in making your decision before buying your oils.

What to ask when purchasing essential oils as described in my previous book, "Emotional Freedom Face-Lift":

- Does the supplier grow and distill their own organic herbs? Are the seeds original, heirloom seeds? Does the supplier distill on the same farm to ensure freshness and potency?

- Are the fragrances subtle, rich, full-body, organic and delicate?

- Does the supplier perform independent lab tests on the essential oils?

- Does the supplier use low pressure and low temperature to distill the plants and preserve the fragile constituents?

- Are the oils labeled 100% pure grade A essential oil aromatherapy totally chemical free?

- Are the oils derived from organic-bio-dynamic plants grown on soil free of pesticides and herbicides to produce the highest bio-chemical qualities?

Can you visit the company's' farms? Are the farms environmentally sustainable?

Probably the most important criteria in choosing a high quality, genuine essential oil is this: can the oils be taken internally- that is, can they be ingested in food, water or capsules? Can they be used intravenously? Simply said: If you can't eat it, then don't wear it and don't smell it!

WHY USE YOUNG LIVING© ESSENTIAL OILS FOR GREENING OUR HOMES

One Word describes this company's oils: **QUALITY**. Young Living is the largest grower of organic essential oils (with over seven privately owned farms) in the world. This company also has the highest and largest selection of quality essential oils on the world market. These products are a cut above organic: They're certified Pure Therapeutic Grade© and distilled without chemical solvents or adulterants.

Young Living essential oils are:

- **NATURAL & PURE** - 100 percent natural, with no artificial ingredients, fragrances or fillers.

- **SAFE** - FDA-approved as GRAS (Generally Regarded As Safe), meaning they can be taken internally or as food additives. Free of pesticides and other chemical residues. No adulterants or solvents used in distillation.

- **POWERFUL** - Standardized active compounds, superfood, fully charged with nutrients

All About Young Living

*The Young Living Mission:
"We honor our stewardship to
champion nature's living energy—
essential oils—by fostering a
community of healing and discovery
while inspiring individuals to wellness,
purpose and abundance."*

Not only does Young Living own its organic herb farms, but they also contract with farmers in other countries to grow plants that meet their high standards – that is Young Living's high standards for therapeutic purposes. Quality control testing of every batch of oil by 2-4 independent laboratories further guarantees that not only are Young Living`s oils, but those acquired from wholesalers around the world, meet the highest standards under the most rigorous testing conditions.

This company has achieved the World standard and is recognized as the world leader in essential oils.

Young Living's quality control protocols are rigorously applied to every batch of oils placed in its warehouse for distribution to customers, arguably a system that is setting the standard for quality control in the aromatherapy industry in the U.S.

Young Living has developed one of the world's largest organic herb farms for the production of therapeutic grade essential oils and owns more than 1,800 acres of organic farmland in Utah and Idaho with over 70,000 square feet of greenhouse space.

Young Living also participates in joint-venture research farms in Provence, France, and Seville, Spain. Recent discoveries in Ecuador have led the company's founder and owner, Dr. Gary Young to operate a farm in Ecuador as well as in Oman. Young Living is one of the few companies in the world that has taken extraordinary pains to preserve all of nature's fragile chemical constituents in essential oils. Young Living is the world's leader in the cultivation, distillation and production of organically grown, guaranteed pure essential oils. Today, Gary Young has expanded his herbal farms worldwide-he's the largest grower and owner in the world with farms in Mona, Utah, St. Maries, Idaho, France as well as Ecuador, Peru and Oman.

Searching for a company that delivers high quality isn't easy-The quality of an essential oil is everything. Low pressure and low temperature are the keys to maintaining the ultimate fragrance and therapeutic value. High pressure, high temperatures, rapid processing and the use of solvents or any other chemical will fracture the oil molecule, destroy the oil's therapeutic value and alter the oil's fragrance and healing qualities. Any chemical, when combined with an essential oil will destroy the effectiveness of the oil's purpose.

An essential oil that is pure, unadulterated, high quality and even therapeutic grade is safe and powerfully effective for people of all ages. But poor quality oil can actually be harmful, especially if used repeatedly on the skin. Oils that have been distilled too quickly or with too much heat and pressure will not have the balanced proportion of components that give an essential oil such safety and effectiveness.

I personally have had the privilege to take part in a number of reforestation initiatives, as well as harvesting herbs on the sustainably-managed Idaho farm. Young Living has set the world standards for healing, therapeutic oils by adhering to their responsible farming guidelines:

Pristine land and virgin soil "The only way you can be sure that land is truly organic is to find untitled land far from the pollution of urban centres." The soil is fortified with minerals, enzymes, manure and mulch.

Carefully selected seeds and planting Seeds are nurtured in greenhouses, so they can adjust to the outside climate and produce the highest quality essential oils. Young Living Essential Oils is the only company dedicated to the **medicinal uses of essential oils** that is able to guarantee essential oil quality from seed to seal.

Organic weed and pest control Young Living practices strict organic farming and does not use synthetic chemicals, pesticides, herbicides or fungicides. A natural blend of essential oils is used to keep weeds in check.

Mountain water irrigation All crops are irrigated using pure mountain water.

Precision harvesting Fields must be harvested at the correct time of year and even time of day in order to optimize oil quality.

Compare that to other essential oil producers, who buy their oils from brokers!

Young Living Therapeutic Grade

"Anyone Can Claim to Be Therapeutic Grade. Only Young Living Can Claim Young Living Therapeutic Grade."

What does Therapeutic Grade mean?

Young Living has created its own standards based on the true medicinal effects of the essential oils in actual therapeutic application. Thus, their standards are even higher than those of the International Organization for Standardization (ISO).

Therapeutic Grade - a term that was coined by Dr. Gary Young the founder, owner of Young Living- to describe his high-quality Young Living essential oils - is the best quality oil that you can purchase—superior to organic oils. There are four grades of essential oils being produced today:

Synthetic or nature-identical oils are created in a laboratory.

Extended or altered oils are fragrance grade.

Natural oils (organic) and certified oils can pass oil-standard tests but may contain just a few therapeutic compounds or none at all.

Therapeutic-grade essential oils are pure, medicinal, steam-distilled essential oils containing all desired therapeutic compounds.

Young Living's Kosher Certification

Young Living Essential Oils' most popular products are kosher-certified! Being kosher-certified means that a product is fit to use in any application in a manner that conforms to the kosher laws rooted in Biblical and Rabbinic traditions. These products and the facilities that produce them have been inspected and found to meet strict kosher requirements.

Distillation of Essential Oils

The key to producing a quality essential oil with all its benefits is to preserve the delicate compounds of the aromatic plant through expert distillation procedures. The proper process of steam distillation—passing steam through the plant material and condensing the steam to separate the oil from the plant—is strictly adhered to with all Young Living essential oils. D. Gary Young has created the world standard to maintain the proper temperature and pressure throughout the distillation process, strictly monitoring the length of time, equipment and batch size. This ensures that the naturally-occurring compounds contained in each essential oil product are of the highest and most consistent bioactive levels.

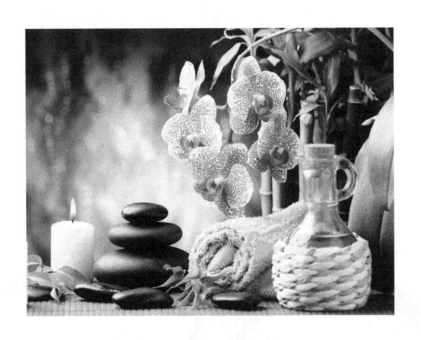

CHAPTER 3:

Healthy Cleaning with Essential Oils including Mold

"Look in the perfumes of flowers and of nature for peace of mind and joy in life"

- Wang Wei, 8th Century A.D.

CHAPTER 3:

One of the last areas you may think to use essential oils is in your cleaning products—especially as cleansers and disinfectants. As we discussed in Chapter 1, most modern cleaning products utilize harmful, toxic chemicals and surfactants (cleansing agents). It is helpful that you know what they are and their potential toxic effects: illness and poisoning of our lands and our wildlife. It's most important to find ways to limit your exposure to these toxins, and instead to learn **safe, effective and healthy alternatives.**

I have personally chosen to use essential oils from the company that is considered today to be the world leader in purity, integrity, potency and efficacy in essential oils— the company that owns, grows, harvests and distills the largest organic herb farms in the world. Young Living has established credibility with eminent scientists and medical professionals worldwide. **The company continually researches and validates their oils' effectiveness and purity, to provide the highest quality product possible as discussed in Chapter 2.**

There are many companies who make claims as to their quality but do not provide information about their quality assurances or procedures. With Young Living, you know who your grower is. When D. Gary Young (owner/founder/CEO of Young Living) brought back 13 essential oils from Europe in 1985, virtually no written information was available about their usage and application. The essential oils that were sold in a few health food and novelty stores were perfume grade, with no suggested therapeutic usage. Young Living set the world standards.

The Thieves Oil© blend, a proprietary combination by Young Living, is **a potent combination of essential oils and a safe, effective start as a cleanser.** The Thieves essential oil blend is one of the more popular cleaning and healing oils that Young Living sells.

INTRODUCING THE THIEVES ESSENTIAL OIL BLEND©

In the battle against harmful germs and rampant mutated, drug-resistant bacterias and superbugs found in our hospitals, homes, offices and now more rampant in our communities, the Thieves line of products from Young Living is a highly effective shield. The Thieves blend provides a full spectrum "overwhelming force" to eradicate pathogens without any harsh chemicals and medicines.

The Thieves Oil Blend was created based on research about four thieves in France who covered themselves with cloves, rosemary and other aromatics while robbing plague victims. It is formulated with highly antiviral, antiseptic, antibacterial and anti-infectious therapeutic-grade essential oils.

Proven effectiveness

Scientists have verified that essential oils kill the deadly Methicillin-Resistant Staphylococcus Aureus (MRSA) superbug, also known as "flesh-eating disease"! In a 2012 study, researchers noted that essential oils have been used for hundreds of years against bacteria, fungi, and viruses. In tests, **four essential oils were found to kill this staph germ: cassia, Peru balsam, red thyme and clove.** The study reported that while this pathogen is resistant to oxacillin and methicillin drugs, it was effectively killed by the essential oils.

The Thieves Oil Blend was researched at Weber State University, where the oils were found to be highly effective in destroying over 99.96 percent of bacteria while preventing mutations.

It is highly effective for:

- Supporting the immune system and good health

- Fighting airborne bacteria and other pathogens

- Eliminating mold and mildew (more on Mold later in this chapter)

- Other studies pertaining to the oils used in the blend showed that:

- Essential oils of **cinnamon, clove,** lemongrass, geranium and thyme were equal or superior to the powerful anti-fungal drug Hexaconzasole.

- The essential oil of cinnamon at a 0.04 percent concentration completely stopped the growth of **35 different fungi, including Aspergillus**— of which infections in the lungs could result in death.

- Clove essential oil, with its primary constituent Eugenol, was found to destroy more than **60 types of bacteria, 15 strains of fungi and several viruses.**

- A solution of .05 percent eugenol from clove oil was sufficient to kill the tuberculosis bacillus.

- Clove oil at only 6 to 8 parts in 10,000 totally inhibited mold and aflatoxin production.

- The essential oils of thyme, origanum, mint, cinnamon, salvia and clove were found to possess the strongest antimicrobial properties among the many agents tested.

Ingredients
The Thieves Oil Blend consists of:

- **Clove** (*Syzygium aromaticum*) – destroys mold, fungus, flu and more. Clove is the highest-scoring ingredient of all those tested for antioxidant capacity on the ORAC scale (with a score of over 10,000,000). **Clove oil is the highest rated antioxidant in the world!**

- **Lemon** *(Citrus limon)* - has antiseptic-like properties, is anti-fungal, antibacterial and contains compounds that amplify immunity. It promotes circulation, leukocyte formation and lymphatic function.

- **Cinnamon** *(Cinnamonum verum)* - destroys MRSA, staphylococcus, fungi and other bacteria.

- **Eucalyptus** *(Eucalyptus radiata)* - a relatively gentle and non-irritating variety that is highly anti-microbial.

- **Rosemary** *(Rosmarinus Officinalis CT cineol)* - anti-fungal and antiseptic as well as being beneficial for helping to restore mental alertness when experiencing fatigue.

For more detail on each of these ingredients, see the Index of Essential Oils.

ESSENTIAL OILS IN MODERN MEDICINE

A number of hospitals in the U.S. are now using Young Living therapeutic essential oils, including Thieves Oil Blend, to prevent and eliminate mold from offices, surgery wards and intensive care units—as well as antiseptics, to treat odors, for relaxation and for various other therapies.

The third largest hospital in the US—the Cleveland Clinic—is now utilizing Young Living Therapeutic standard essential oils for complimentary therapies. The hospital is diffusing the revolutionary Young Living essential oils at nursing stations, in their PACU, physicians' lounges and in some offices. The Cleveland Clinic Healing Services Team would never even entertain the idea of using any other essential oil in their hospital. They know that the Young Living Essential Oils will not only provide them with the level of quality that they expect, but the oils are always consistent in their formulations and thus will ensure the best possible outcomes for their patients.

One of the most prestigious partners with Young living is the **Beth Israel Medical Center** in New York. Woodson Merrel, M.D.—Director of Integrative Medicine at Beth Israel—has partnered with Young Living and **uses only Young Living oils in hospital cancer wards as well as in supportive care facilities.** Dr. Merrell is a high profile medical doctor whose expertise includes mind-body therapies, acupuncture, botanical therapies, nutrition and nutraceuticals, homeopathy and indigenous healing systems. (See Dr. Merrel share his views in this online video: http://youtu.be/6pU72bqSXHk)

Donna Karan is a famous fashion designer who introduced Young Living essential oils to the Urban Zen Foundation, and eventually to the Beth Israel Medical Center. As Karan points out in her interview, hospitals have "some of the most wicked smells, along with a lot of toxicities." She chose Young

Living oils "to have the aromatherapy that truly works." (Watch the video online: http://youtu.be/Bas5VRcLmgc)

The **Children's National Medical Center** is a pediatric hospital in Washington, DC and a leader in developing innovative new treatments for childhood illnesses. The local NBC news affiliate reports on the innovative ways that essential oils are used in the center. The Children's National Medical Center chooses Young Living Essential Oils to help in pain management because Young Living's oils are Therapeutic Grade. (Watch the report online: http://youtu.be/elc4W3JUJlc)

Another holistic center that has embraced complimentary therapies with Young Living oils is the **Oaklawn Medical Group in Albion, Michigan**. Many of Oaklawn's daily operations and treatments come from nutritional therapists, massage therapists, naturopathic practitioners, and other practitioners of complementary techniques. Currently, the center uses Young Living Therapeutic Grade Essential Oils to strengthen the immune system of patients and treat specific health issues with aromatherapy and Raindrop Technique massage.

It's reassuring to know that major hospitals are utilizing these essential oils that have been shown to possess the strongest antimicrobial properties in the plant kingdom warding off microbes, toxic smells, chemical toxins and many more attributes.

INTRODUCING THE THIEVES HOUSEHOLD CLEANER©

The Thieves Oil blend is very effective and an all-time favorite combination of oils. Now you can get more out of its power by using the new **Thieves Household Cleaner** for tough jobs.

The Thieves Household Cleaner boasts the most effective 100 percent plant- and mineral-based ingredients available:

- Vegetable-based surfactants like alkyl polyglucoside, compliant with Green Seal and EPA Design for Environment standards.

- Biodegradable cutting agents like sodium methyl 2-sulfolurate and disodium 2-sulfolaurate, from renewable sources.

- Active ingredients like tetrasodium glutamate diacetate, readily biodegradable and derived from food-approved amino acids.

- The all-natural cleansing and disinfecting power of therapeutic-grade Thieves and lemon essential oils. All of the ingredients that make up this new formulation are ecologically friendly, come from sustainable sources and have biodegradable properties; none of them are petroleum-based.

In addition, every one of these ingredients received a **_Green rating_** from the Environmental Working Group and uses ecologically responsible packaging, meaning that they're **good for you, good for the planet, and good for the community.**

Every product in the Thieves line has been infused with pure, therapeutic-grade essential oils. Great care has been taken to ensure that each essential oil contained in Young Living's products meets the highest standard for purity and potency.

Thieves Household Cleaner is highly concentrated and can be diluted for any size of job, with dilution ratios conveniently listed on the label. Just one bottle offers countless ways to clean—from laundry and dishes to floors, counters tops, bathrooms, carpets, upholstery and much more. Thieves is also available in a convenient 64-ounce value size.

With more of the Thieves oil blend and lemon essential oils, the new Thieves Household Cleaner disinfects and cleanses better than ever!!

What is "Plant-Based"?

Tracy Gibbs, PhD consulted with Young Living on the development of the new Thieves household cleaner. The term "plant-based" can cause some confusion, so Young Living talked with Tracy about what it means to have a 100 percent plant- and mineral-based formula:

"Basically, if you trace any chemical back to its origin, it all comes from nature at some point; the key is in the extraction process," Tracy says. "Plant-based ingredients are

those extracted from the source without the use of synthetic chemicals—typically by using water or ethanol. **When you use plant-based, biodegradable products you have zero impact on the environment.** *It's important to use a natural household cleaner because it's what you do every day that matters. That's what determines your health and where being environmentally friendly counts the most."*

Ecologically responsible packaging

Thieves cleaner's packaging is recyclable, with an added option to purchase the standard 14-ounce bottle, or a new 64-ounce economy size. We encourage you to buy in bulk and do your part to cut down on packaging waste and production emissions.

MOLD: HIDDEN HEALTH DANGERS
Why is Mold a Danger?

Mold issues are probably one of the most common, hidden and most toxic home problems. Molds are microscopic fungi that produce tiny spores to reproduce by landing on a damp spot digesting whatever they are growing on in order to survive. They belong to the Fungi kingdom. Molds gradually destroy the things they grow on, no matter what it is: building materials, furnishings, paper, carpet, walls, foods, wood and people.

They are found everywhere in the environment both indoor and outdoor. In fact, all the spores need to colonize and grow is moisture. They are 'neurotoxic mycotoxins' (chemicals that are produced by the spores as they live and grow called mycotoxins) and cause serious health problems including psychiatric disorders and cancer. Exposure pathways for these microscopic mycotoxins can include inhalation, ingestion, or skin contact. The Environmental Protection Agency (EPA) website is replete with information on Mold. http://www.epa.gov/mold/moldresources.html

Moisture control is the key to mold control.

- More than 200 mycotoxins have been identified from common molds and many more remain to be identified. (EPA) Some of the molds that are known to produce mycotoxins are commonly found in moisture-damaged buildings. There are a variety of toxic molds; most dangerous being toxic Black Mold, called Stachybotrys. **Stachybotrys** (black mold), **Aspergillus** and **Cladosporium** are three of the most dangerous and commonly found indoor toxic molds.

- **"Growth of mold in buildings is no longer just a cosmetic problem but is a potential threat to human health."** — American Industrial Hygiene Association (AIHA).

Researchers at the U.S. EPA (Environmental Protection Agency) estimated that 50 percent of homes contain mold-friendly dampness or fungi, which raises risk of **respiratory disease** by up to 50 percent. Particularly susceptible are pregnant women, infants, the elderly and those with pre-existing health conditions.

A University survey of 160 homes found mold in all of them, and in places most people wouldn't think to look.

After surveying 160 homes in seven U.S. cities, Kelly A. Reynolds of the University of Arizona, Tucson, found that ***100 percent of the homes tested positive*** for mold on some inside surface. (Kathleen Doheny: Health Day News Reporter)

In 1999, the Mayo Clinic concluded that 96 percent of chronic sinus infections are caused by fungi. Symptoms can include headaches; nose, eye and throat irritation; nosebleeds and coughs; skin irritation and respiratory infections. *Asthma rates* have more than doubled since 1980; mold is an *asthma trigger*. In one recent study, **infants exposed to household mold were more likely to develop asthma by the age of seven.**

Mold is a highly common cause of *allergic symptoms*. Toxic black mold Stachybotrys—found in homes, offices and school environments—has been linked to *fatal pulmonary disorders.*

A groundbreaking public health study at Brown University has found **a connection between damp, moldy homes and depression.** The study, an analysis of data from nearly 6,000 European adults, is the largest investigation into the association between mold and mood. Lead researcher Edward Shenassa said the findings, published in the *American Journal of Public Health*, came as a complete surprise. "We thought that once we statistically accounted for factors that could clearly contribute to depression—things like employment status and crowding—we would see any link vanish," said Shenassa, the lead author of the study and an associate professor in the Department of Community Health at Brown University. "But the opposite was true. **We found a solid association between depression and living in a damp, moldy home.**"

Molds are toxins and some research has indicated that these toxins can affect the nervous system or the immune system or impede the function of the frontal cortex, the part of the brain that plays a part in impulse control, memory, problem solving, sexual behavior, socialization and spontaneity. This study is another reminder in the importance of eliminating toxic mold.

North Americans spend on average 90 percent of their lives indoors; Is it any wonder that there's a growing public concern about the impact of mold on human health? Look at the number of symptoms caused by mold exposure: and further on, the psychiatric symptoms:

- Allergies

- Fatigue (chronic, excessive, or continued)

- Asthma

- Flu symptoms (chronic)

- Bleeding lungs

- General malaise

- Breathing difficulties

- Sudden hair loss

- Cancer

- Headaches

- Hemorrhagic pneumonitis

- Central nervous system problems

- Dermatitis

- Recurring colds

- Skin rash

- Eye and vision problems

- Diarrhea

- Chronic coughing or coughing with blood

Other rare symptoms:

- At the University of Texas MD Anderson Cancer Center, approximately 15-20% of patients with leukemia die of *fungal leukemia* caused most frequently by the species Aspergillus.

- In patients with leukemia 15-30% of deaths are caused by _refractory fungal infections_ such as Aspergillus, one of the most dangerous indoor molds.

EPA and its Science Advisory Board (SAB) have consistently ranked indoor air pollution among the top four environmental risks to public health.

- Several of the **Cladosporium** spores are known to cause skin lesions, keratitis, nail fungus, sinusitis, asthma, and pulmonary infections.

- Prolonged exposure to **Cladosporium** can cause edema, bronchio spasms and emphysema.

Dr. James Schaller, a medical doctor, psychiatrist, an author with 27 books and 27 peer-reviewed journal articles and a certified mold remediator and investigator treats mold illness. He combines his expertise in his clinical work with alternative approaches to health conditions. Dr. Schaller is a full-time researcher and part-time clinician working as a pioneer in mold illness. He identified a number of psychiatric symptoms related to toxic mold exposures that are outlined below.

- Headaches
- **Poor memory**
- Trouble concentrating
- **Trouble learning**

- Trouble finding words
- **Disorientation**
- Seizures
- Trouble speaking fast
- Trouble with understanding fast
- Trembling
- Vocal or Motor Tics
- **Serotonin changes**
- Poor insight
- Poor insight into illness
- **Decreased productivity**
- **Unable to process trauma or interpersonal pain**
- **Mood swings**
- **Mania**
- Irritability
- **Impulsivity**
- Depression
- Anxiety

HIDE AND SEEK: MOLD LOCATIONS

- Within a home or building, moisture can be in the form of excessive humidity (e.g., in a bathroom or laundry room), condensation (e.g., resulting from 'cold spots' due to poor insulation around windows), or seeping water (e.g., from a leaky roof or pipe).

- Newer homes and buildings are not immune from moisture; in fact, they are often more prone to mold. Buildings are now made so air tight that the pollutants produced in the building accumulate and have no way to escape.

- You can smell mold in cinemas, locker rooms and other dark, damp places where molds thrive.

- Toxic mold can be inside walls, under tubs, behind appliances etc. and you may not be able to see it.

"Excessive dampness influences whether mold, as well as bacteria, dust mites and other such agents are present and thrive indoors". Institute of Medicine, May 25, 2004

FOODS too - *Aspergillus niger* a fungus, is one of the most common species of the genus *Aspergillus*. It causes black mold on certain types of fruit and vegetables and is a common contaminant of food.

Important points to Remember:

- **What makes you sick is usually not the organisms themselves, but the airborne toxins and allergens they produce.** Many of the chemical solutions in the clean-up can cause just as many problems.

- Most products that claim to kill fungi – whether bleach-based, ammonia-based, or otherwise – do so by overexposing the microorganism to **toxic chemical substances.**

- These same chemicals are poisonous to humans and animals.

- As a result, the fumes and residue that these products generate during and after use pose health risks to users and building occupants.

- Thus- Keeping mold at bay requires vigilance along with the proper cleaning solutions.

- It's critical to clean areas before mold has a chance to build up.

Bleach, ozone and other biocides are not recommended solutions.

As we discussed in Chapter 1, Chlorine bleach is toxic. When mixed with molds, it can be deadly.

According to the EPA, **the use of bleach, or any other chemical or biocide that kills organisms is not recommended to clean up mold.** This statement is directly posted on the EPA website, advising no bleach: "The use of a chemical or biocide that kills organisms such as mold (chlorine bleach, for example) is not recommended as a routine practice during mold cleanup."

Commonly used chemicals do not effectively kill molds. For example, active fungal growth on a surface may produce a spore density of 1 million spores per square inch. Treating this site with a biocide that has an effectiveness of 99.9 percent would still leave an estimated 1,000 viable spores per square inch. Dr. Edward Close (an environmental engineer) points out how the commonly used chemicals for mold clean up cause other problems for the homeowner –

Here are a few that he suggests on his website http://moldrx4u.com:

- Mold usually returns in less than 24 hours after using bleach.

- Cleaning stirs up mold spores and puts them into the air, creating more mold related health problems and allergic reactions.

- Bleach only treats the surface. It does not kill or eliminate airborne mold spores.

- Bleach is ineffective and not recommended for use on porous surfaces such as concrete, wood, wallpaper, sheetrock, grout, books, clothing

- Chlorine Gas, released by mixing bleach with any acid, may be lethal.

- Chlorine particles, according to some reports,

may bio-accumulate in the Thyroid leading to reduced thyroid function and possibly thyroid cancer.

So how do you destroy toxic mold quickly and keep it from coming back?

NOVEL WAY: Eliminate mold and stay healthy with Thieves

Thieves Household Cleaner is a revolutionary, natural and organic way to remove mold and fungus growth using essential oils. It's a 100 percent pure, organic, biodegradable blend of plant extracts that is so safe and non-toxic that it is used and approved as a food supplement.

A 1997 study at Weber State University demonstrated the killing power of these amazing oils against airborne microorganisms:

- After 10 minutes, the number of gram positive *Micrococcus luteus* organisms was reduced by 82 percent.

- After 12 minutes, *M. luteus* were reduced by 90 percent.

- **After 20 minutes, *M. luteus* were reduced by 99.3 percent.**

- *Pseudomonas aeruginosa* showed a kill rate of **99.96 percent after just 12 minutes.**

Dr. Edward Close is an environmental engineer, environmental science expert and environmental advisor to Fortune 500 companies. He discovered & proved that Thieves essential oil destroys toxic mold and keeps it from coming back. Astoundingly, he found that Thieves creates **100 percent remediation of mold!** Even better, these same organic therapeutic essential oils can be used internally and topically for colds, flus and other health-related issues. His website outlines his discoveries, as well as his book: *"Natures' Mold Rx: The Non-Toxic Solution to Toxic Mold."*

In 2005, Dr. Close was asked to do third-party sampling for mold in an apartment complex that had been flooded, evacuated, and later put up for sale. The buyer, who was renovating the apartments, had paid a company to use the strongest products they knew of—a hospital disinfectant. Yet Dr. Close's sampling showed that either the product had not killed the mold or that the mold had already re-established itself.

After much urging by his wife to do the study, Dr. Close diffused Thieves essential oil in the apartments for a 24-hour period. **The research project yielded astonishing results!** See them explained in this online video by Dr. Close: http://youtu.be/28fez0T17cM

In another instance, 10,667 stachybotrys mold spores were identified in a per cubic meter area. After diffusing Thieves essential oil for 48 hours, Dr Close retested. Only thirteen stachybotrys remained. Similarly, 75,000 stachybotrys mold spores were identified in a sample of sheetrock. After 72 hours of diffusing, no stachybotrys mold spores remained.

Disappearing Toxic Mold Spores:

- 10,667 to 13 in 48 hours
- 75,000 to 0 in 72 hours

Dr. Edward Close discovered and proved that Thieves essential Oil destroys toxic mold and keeps it from returning— in other words it's ***100 percent long term remediation!***

According to Dr. Close there is no other remediation that is available that gives such outstanding results: "My research and the scientific data collected clearly demonstrate Young Living's Thieves Oil Blend and Thieves Household Cleaner are the ***BEST*** **treatment** options available today for eliminating Toxic Mold from your life."

One of the most important findings of the more than 20 case studies that were conducted by Dr. Edward Close is simply this:

* diffusing the essential oil blend not only destroyed the mold spores, but also removed mold spores, dead and alive, from the air. This in itself is a very important finding.

* There is indirect evidence from these case studies that suggest that exposure to the toxins released by these molds may also be eliminated by diffusing the essential oil blend.

There is no other product that is all organic and biodegradable in remediating toxic mold that can also be taken internally for:

- health conditions (colds, sore throats, flu)

- boosting your immune system

- oral health

- baking and food supplementation

- balancing your blood sugar

--all at the same time!

MOLD REMEDIATION
How do you know there is a Mold Problem?

1) By Smell- this is usually a tell tale sign (often noticed in locker rooms, cottages, bathrooms etc.) to take action

2) By Visual signs- often Mold will appear in shower stalls, refrigerators, ceilings etc.

3) By people not feeling well in the area- so suspect hidden mold – look for leaks, too much humidity

4) Test with a humidity sensor

5) Call a mold remediation expert to test your space– as Mold can be hidden behind the drywall etc.

Further steps for at- home Mold Clean-up is presented in Chapter 7.

KITCHENS: GREENING YOUR FOOD

There are over 76 million cases of food poisoning per year, with 80 percent caused at home. We have answers to help keep your kitchen green clean and food-safe. **Many essential oils are disinfectants and antiseptics, and will ward off salmonella, *E. coli* and other pathogens.**

According to Environmental Working Group's latest March 2013 report, superbugs are on the rise—and they're in supermarkets! Tests of ground raw turkey conducted in 2006 found that 82 percent of *E. coli* bacteria (responsible for 6 million infections a year) were antibiotic-resistant. In 2011, federal scientists determined that **74 percent of the salmonella bacteria on raw chicken were antibiotic-resistant, up from less than 50 percent in 2002.**

Protecting yourself is easy with essential oils, and they're proven to be effective. For the past decade, a series of studies in food microbiology have been testing the efficacy of essential oils for food storage purposes as well as food preservation. These studies were conducted at the Université du Québec's Research Laboratories in Sciences Applied to Food, headed by lead researcher, Professor Monique Lacriox and were published in the peer-reviewed *Journal of Agricultural and Food Chemistry* in 2004 and 2005.

One such study applied an essential oils mix containing oregano oil on beef. Results showed that **the use of film** containing essential oils significantly reduced the growth of pathogenic bacteria, including *E. coli,* as compared to meat that was non-treated. The researchers concluded: "The application of bioactive films on meat surfaces ... showed that film containing oregano oil was the most effective against both bacterias."

In another study, the authors assert that essential oils and their components are active against a wide variety of microorganisms, including pathogenic Gram-negative bacteria. Several oils were tested for efficacy with the Pseudomonas putida strain. **Seven essential oils were shown to have strong antimicrobial activity against P. putida, while ten other oils also showed a high antimicrobial activity at a different dilution rate.**

These studies allow the researchers to demonstrate that essential oils have real use as natural protectors of our food and health. The authors point out that essential oils have 'long served as flavoring agents in food and beverages, and due to their versatile content of antimicrobial compounds, they possess potential as natural agents for food preservation'.

In fact, from ancient times, essential oils have been used as food preservatives, disinfectants, antiseptics, and much more; science is re-discovering their use today. Studies are showing that essential oils are a must for every kitchen sink, countertop and cutting board.

Bathrooms: Go green, refresh and cleanse safely

Your bathroom may contain "potentially" toxic, harmful, poisonous and even carcinogenic ingredients. Look at your toothpaste, shampoo, mouthwash, shaving cream and moisturisers! Many commonly used products contain potentially harmful ingredients, which may penetrate the skin and build up in vital organs and tissues. **The bathroom is one of the most toxic rooms in the house for most American families**.

Toxins found in typical household bathroom products:

- **Aluminum** - A metallic element used extensively in the manufacture of aircraft components, prosthetic devices, and as an ingredient in antiperspirants, antacids, and antiseptics. Aluminium has been linked to Alzheimer's disease.

- **Animal fat (tallow)** - A type of animal tissue made up of oily solids or semisolids that are water-insoluble esters of glycerol with fatty acids. Animal fats and lye are the chief ingredients in bar soap, a cleansing and emulsifying product that may act as a breeding ground for bacteria.

- **Propylene glycol** - A cosmetic form of mineral oil found in automatic brake and hydraulic fluid, and industrial antifreeze. In skin and hair care products, propylene glycol works as a humectant, which is a substance that retains the moisture content of skin or cosmetic products by preventing the escape of moisture or water. Material Safety Data Sheets (MSDS) warn users to avoid skin contact with propylene glycol, as this strong skin irritant can cause liver abnormalities and kidney damage.

- **Sodium lauryl sulfate (SLS) - Harsh detergents and wetting agents used in garage floor cleaners, engine degreasers, and automotive cleaning products are also found in toothpaste, soaps and shampoos.** SLS is well-known in the scientific community as a common skin irritant. It is rapidly absorbed and retained in the eyes, brain, heart, and liver, which may result in harmful long-term effects. SLS could retard healing, cause cataracts in adults and keep children's eyes from developing properly.

These chemical toxins are only a few found in an average home's bathroom. Stop polluting your body! See Chapters 7 through 9 for safe, effective solutions.

Are your clothes *really* clean?

What's lurking on your freshly washed clothes?

You'll be horrified when you discover what's showing up in your clothes, towels and sheets, freshly laundered in your own home's washing machine or your local laundromat. The chemicals in laundry detergent leave a residue that threatens you and your family's health in a way you may never have. Dr. Mercola's articles on this topic have been revealing more of these toxic laundry compounds.

Do you know how safe your detergent is? **Most laundry detergents contain a potentially toxic brew of chemicals that can leave residues behind on your clothing, be absorbed by your skin or be released into the air you breathe.**

Dryer sheets coat all your clothes with a layer of toxic chemicals. When you wear those clothes, your body moisture causes those chemicals to come into contact with your skin and be absorbed directly into your bloodstream. It's an easy way to poison your system with cancer-causing chemicals.

The laundry room is also highly toxic: The room is exposed to the same chemical perfumes released by the laundry detergent and dryer sheets.

Our ancestors scented their laundry to have fresh, clean-smelling clothes. They would dry their clothes on rosemary or lavender bushes to scent them. It was also popular to lay sprigs of lavender between the clean linens in cupboards to keep them fresh smelling.

Lavender is known for its fresh scent and melaleuca for its disinfecting power. Stop the "Bounce" and scent your clothes naturally, the way Mother Nature intended!

What potentially toxic and carcinogenic chemicals are you wearing?

Listed below are just some of the toxic and potential cancer-causing chemicals found in typical laundry detergents that can not only cause you harm, but raise havoc in the environment as well. These harsh chemicals can build up in your clothes and eventually penetrate your skin. Detergent makers are not required by law to list these ingredients.

- **Sodium lauryl sulfate (SLS)** – Chemical foaming agent known as a surfactant. Studies have linked use of this chemical to a variety of health issues from skin irritation to organ toxicity.

- **Dioxane (1,4-dioxane)** – The majority of top laundry detergent brands contain this synthetic petrochemical, a known carcinogen. This is a byproduct contaminant of the manufacturing process and is not required to be listed on product labels.

- **Linear alky benzene sulfonates (LAS)** – Synthetic petrochemicals that biodegrade slowly making them an environmental hazard. Benzene may cause cancer in humans and animals.

- **Nonylphenol ethoxylate (NPE)** – Petrochemical surfactant banned in the EU and Canada. May cause liver and kidney damage. Biodegradable, but biodegrades into more toxic substances.

- **Petroleum distillates (aka napthas)** – Derived from synthetic crude oil, linked to cancer and lung and mucous membrane damage.

- **Artificial fragrances** – Linked to various toxic effects on fish and mammals, and can cause allergies, skin and eye irritation to humans.

- **Phosphates** – Used to prevent dirt from settling back into clothes after being washed. Can stimulate growth of marine plants that trigger unbalanced ecosystems.

Dangers of 1,4-dioxane

1,4-dioxane is a synthetic petrochemical carcinogen, created when laundry detergents and other cleaning products are cheaply manufactured using ethoxylation (a short-cut industrial process in which ethylene oxide is added to fatty acid alcohols to give them detergent properties).

In 2010, Green Patriot Working Group and the Organic Consumers Association published the results of a study on 1,4 dioxane levels in laundry detergents. About two thirds of the detergents tested contained 1,4 dioxane. Thirteen of them were popular brands, one of which had levels as high as 55 ppm.

The report points out that the **1,4 dioxane in laundry detergent is particularly harmful: the chemical binds easily to water and remains there.** It is not easily removed from water even with purification or filtration. **Numerous water supplies across the country have been found to be tainted with 1,4 dioxane.**

And since 1,4-dioxane is considered a byproduct, it's technically recognized as a contaminant and doesn't require listing on the product label.

1,4-dioxane:

- is considered a carcinogen by the State of California

- has been found to be potentially toxic to your brain and nervous system

- potentially causes issues with your kidneys, liver, and respiratory system

- due to its lack of effective biodegradability, is an increasing threat to waterways.

AIR FRESHENING

We have already seen a few chemicals most often used in air fresheners, such as formaldehyde (linked to cancer) and phthalates (also carcinogenic). Others, like acetone (a blood, heart, gastrointestinal, liver, kidney, skin, respiratory, brain and nervous system toxin), are also utilized in popular metered air fresheners. Another is benzene, known to cause leukemia in humans...xylene, toluene, styrene...but **there are so many toxic chemicals in air fresheners that the list can become overwhelming. Keep it simple: don't pollute your air with commercially fragranced products!**

Homes, offices, lobbies, hotels, even nurseries are bombarded with these toxic, synthetic smells used as air "fresheners" or room "deodorizers": **plug-ins, sticks, wicks, mists, aerosols, carpet cleaners, scented candles and even scented stones.**

Many are highly toxic and cause a range of diseases when inhaled (for example, inhaling formaldehyde in small amounts can cause coughing, a sore throat, respiratory and eye problems and is linked to cancer particularly in the nasal cavity). **Exposure to so-called "air fresheners"—as little as once a week—can greatly increase your odds of developing asthma and can contribute to an increase in pulmonary diseases.**

A nationwide survey found that people with high blood levels of the chemical 1,4 dichlorobenze, which is commonly found in popular air fresheners, were more likely to experience a decline in lung function.

In 2007, The Natural Resources Defense Council discovered and reported that most chemical air "fresheners" contained variable amounts of phthalates. **None of the air fresheners that were tested listed phthalates on their labels. Phthalates are known to interfere with hormone and testosterone production. Children and unborn babies are particularly vulnerable to the toxins. (See Chapter 1)**

TIME MAGAZINE (SEPTEMBER 24, 2007) WENT ON TO REPORT:

"The U.S. Food and Drug Administration has no regulations on the use of phthalates, does not require the labeling of phthalate content on products and does not consider the quantities to which people are exposed to be harmful."

Yet watch enough TV commercials, reports TIME, and one gets the sense that Americans are obsessed with air fresheners. **What sort of toxic chemicals—and at what levels—are we pumping into our homes?**

Create your own air fresheners and avoid adding terrible toxins to your space. See chapter 7 for delightful, natural and Real Green air freshener recipes!

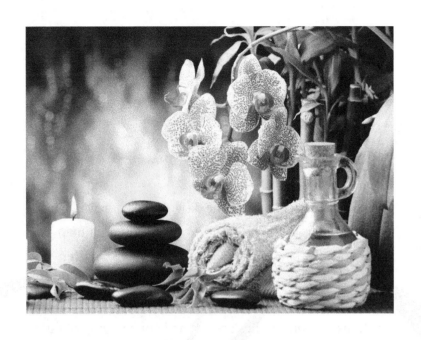

CHAPTER 4:

Energize your home with healing frequencies

"Concerning matter, we have been all wrong. What we have called matter is energy, whose vibration has been so lowered as to be perceptible to the senses. There is no matter."

- Albert Einstein

CHAPTER 4:

WE ARE ENERGY

Quantum physicists over the last 30 years have focused on how energy works and how it affects human life. It is known that **energy always precedes matter,** and that matter accounts for only 2 percent of the universe. We don't often stop to think about it, but our spirit, thoughts, emotions and our bodies are all made of energy—vibrating at a specific frequency like a musical note. Welcome to the world of quantum physics.

I have found quantum physics to be an intriguing area of study: I, like you, am an energy system. When physicists look at matter, they describe it as condensed light. Pythagoras once said 2500 years ago, that "A stone is frozen music" and a modern day physicist David Bohm stated that "A rock is frozen light"! As we learn to utilize these understandings we can create our 'heaven on earth' in our living spaces more efficiently and evolve to higher states as energy beings.

You and I and everything around us are pure energy— light in its most beautiful and intelligent composition.

Our own energy field is connected to the universal energy field. One of the key concepts in quantum physics is that we are one with our universe and that we are mysteriously connected together by an invisible energy that journalist Lynne McTaggart calls "the Field". Some physicists have even referred to it as the Mind of God. We, as human energy beings, are spirit and soul entities: spiritual beings having a physical body experience. As physicist William Tiller states, 'we are all spirits having a physical experience as we go down the river of life'.

"Spirit drives this bio-bodysuit vehicle (our physical body)! After all, 99.999% of all physical 'matter' consists of vacuum, with BIG spaces between electrons and nucleus. The energy potential, or latent energy, stored in one single Hydrogen atom is equivalent to one trillion times all the energy in our universe! If our consciousness could interact with the vacuum, we could have some very BIG effects. We'll be able to use the physics of the vacuum to get to the stars." William Tiller http://www.tiller.org/

Fritz-Albert Popp, a German biophysicist, is also an author of eight books and more than 150 scientific journal articles and studies that address basic questions of theoretical physics, biology and complementary medicine. Popp made the first extensive physical analysis of "biophotons," or units of light emitted by living things. Popp proposed that **all living things emit light energy**. These particles of light, with no mass, transmit information within and between cells. Popp's work shows that DNA in living cells stores and releases photons and also exchanges signals such as electromagnetic waves or matter, creating "biophotonic emissions" that may hold the key to illness and health.

All living cells of plants, animals and human beings emit biophotons, which cannot be seen by the naked eye but can be measured by special equipment developed by German researchers.

Popp and his team discovered that **without photons, chemical reactions are not possible. In other words, 'light makes the world go round'.** In one of his experiments, Popp and his colleagues discovered something remarkable. When the number of emissions in one part of the body increased or decreased, so did emissions in other parts of the body.

We are made up of a cluster of ever-changing energy in the form of electrons, neutrons, photons and so on. Every physical atom floats in a sea of what Descartes called "subtle matter"—the energy that makes up most of what we perceive. Dr. **Deepak Chopra author, medical doctor also made a similar statement like Tiller: "We are 99.999999 percent empty space."**

Every nerve impulse and every cell in our body is an electromagnetic frequency current. We are energy that is constantly changing beneath the surface; you and I have the power to shape that energy with our powerful minds.

Now, leading-edge research is suggesting that the "empty" space within and between atoms is not empty at all. **In fact, the empty space between atoms is so lively with energy that one cubic centimeter—about the size of a marble—contains more energy than all the solid matter in the entire known universe!**

"Energy is all there is."

- Albert Einstein

RAISE YOUR VIBRATION

Illnesses and negative emotions actually **vibrate to a lower frequency**. In his book *Power vs. Force*, David Hawkins developed a "Map of Consciousness" that outlines unknown aspects of consciousness in relationship to one's emotional and spiritual development. Hawkins tested the human body's energetic response to a range of emotions and energies. Negative emotions showed a lower range. **With each progressive rise in the level of consciousness, the "frequency" or "vibration" of energy increased. Higher consciousness radiates a beneficial and healing effect on the world, verifiable in the human muscle response that stays strong in the presence of love and truth.** In contrast, non–true or negative energy fields which "calibrate" below the level of integrity induce a weak muscle response.

To find joy and raise your consciousness, you can **raise your vibration frequency toward the level of love and truth. My goal is to inspire you so that you and our entire human family can reach heights of deeper insights and inner gifts of greatness and potential.** In that practice, the use of essential oils can immensely help to elevate you quickly along with focused intention.

Scientists in the area of natural healing, inspired by the possibility of raising the body's frequency, have conducted extensive research to discover more natural ways to increase the body's vibration. This led to the discovery of the electrical frequencies in essential oils.

The discovery was made when **patients who diffused oils in their homes felt better**. It only took seconds for some patients to feel calmer and less anxious. Certain oils acted almost immediately; others made their effects felt within 1-3 minutes. This discovery led to more remarkable research linking essential oils and energetic vibration.

ESSENTIAL OILS HAVE ELECTRICAL FREQUENCIES!

Clinical research shows that **essential oils have the highest frequency of any natural substance known to humans—** thus having the ability to create an environment in which microbes cannot survive. Lower depressed feelings and negative attitudes can be positively affected with the application of essential oils: They carry a higher frequency range, resulting in a positive change of attitude, mood and/ or spirit.

It's also interesting to note that, based on biophotonic principles, essential oils can be thought of captured light or photons pulsing their own musical note.

The electrical frequency of oils was discovered in 1992 by Bruce Tainio, of Tainio Technology in Washington. Tainio developed new equipment to measure the bio-frequency of humans and foods. He used his bio-frequency monitor to determine the relationship between frequency and disease and later, in collaboration with D. Gary Young, tested the electrical frequencies of essential oils. Below are some of his findings, as presented by Young in his book *Aromatherapy, The Essential Beginning*:

- Processed foods/canned food   0 to 15 MHz

- Dry herbs   12-22 MHz

- Fresh produce   15 to 22 MHz

- Fresh herbs   20-27 MHz

- Essential Oils   47 MHz-320MHz

- The frequency of rose oil is the highest of any substance measured, at 320MHZ.

- Distilled water with 2 drops of peppermint oil added to it had a frequency of 78MHz.

- Distilled water with lemon oil measured at 76 MHz.

- Tap water measured at 32MHz.

Following is a partial list of the frequencies of Young Living essential oil **proprietary blends**, as measured by Bruce Tainio. Young Living is the only company that has ever measured the frequency of essential oils.

- Abundance   78 MHz

- Acceptance   102 MHz

- Aroma Siez   64 MHz

- Awaken   89 MHz

- Brain Power   78 MHz

- Christmas Spirit   104 MHz

- Citrus Fresh   90 MHz

- Clarity   101 MHz

- Di-Gize   102 MHz

- Dragon Time   72 MHz

- Dream Catcher   98 MHz

- Endo Flex   138 MHz

- En-R-Gee   106 MHz

- Envision   90 MHz

- Exodus II   180 MHz

- Forgiveness   192 MHz

- Gathering   99 MHz

- Gentle Baby   152 MHz

- Grounding   140 MHz

- Harmony   101 MHz

- Hope   98 MHz

- Humility   88 MHz

- Immupower   89 MHz

NEW RESEARCH: THE VIBRATION THEORY

Since 1996, Luca Turin has been the leading proponent of **the vibration theory of olfaction.**

Olfaction is the sense of smell. This sense is mediated by specialized sensory cells of the nasal cavity of vertebrates, and, by analogy, sensory cells of the antennae of invertebrates. Turin proposes that **a molecule's smell character is due to its vibrational frequency in the infrared range.** The theory is opposed to the more widely accepted shape theory, which states that a molecule's particular smell is due to a 'lock and key' mechanism by which a scent molecule fits into olfactory receptors in the nasal epithelium.

That is to say: **Do certain things smell good or bad because of the shape of the molecules? Or are we really sensing their vibrational energy?**

The news website *Nature* published an article about a study that supported Turin's theory: "A controversial theory of how we smell, which claims that our fine sense of odour depends on quantum mechanics, has been given the thumbs up by a team of physicists."

The vibration theory received more support from a 2004 paper published in the journal *Organic Biomolecular Chemistry*, which showed that odor descriptions in the olfaction literature correlate more strongly with vibrational frequency than with molecular shape.

How does this all measure up when it comes to your home or your business? **As soon as you begin to use the therapeutic essential oils, you add to your home's frequencies and alter disharmonious energies—as well as neutralizing the pathogens. By this addition alone, you can create safe, happy, joyful and healing spaces!**

For example, the essential oil of lemon myrtle (*Backhousia citriodora*), when taken internally, boosts the body's natural defenses and can also be used as a cleansing agent to purify household surfaces.

Aromatically, lemon myrtle has a powerful lemon scent, even stronger than lemon essential oil. The fresh aroma is uplifting and refreshing, which helps to clear the mind, enhancing concentration or promoting a peaceful night's sleep.

By using essential oils in your home, you can begin to create your "heaven on earth", making your spaces sacred, pure, safe and welcoming.

NATIVE AMERICAN CLEANSING: ANOTHER WAY TO RAISE FREQUENCIES

Since we are talking about creating a safe and energetically healthy space in your home or office, it is important for me to include **a very easy and quick way of cleansing the space, often called "smudging". Smudging is a Native American method to cleanse a person, place or object of negative energies, influences or spirits.**

Smudging usually involves the burning of a sacred plant, then either passing an object through the resulting smoke, or fanning the smoke around while walking through a space. This procedure is often done with a sage smudge stick, though you can use another herb.

- Sage - Cleanses and transmutes all residual negative energy.

- Lavender - Soothes you and your home after heavy energy releases.

- Sweet grass - Restores the flow of Light in your home.

Though the procedure usually involves the burning of a sage bundle, you can substitute by making a smudge aerosol bottle that contains equal parts of Sage essential oil with grain alcohol and ½ cup of distilled water.

First, apply essential oils of Valor on your feet and Sacred Frankincense or Palo Santo on your shoulders while offering a silent prayer or intention of peace and harmony in your space.

Crack a window in each room of your home. Walk around each room, being unemotional, while saying loudly and firmly, as if you were in prayer or mediation, these words:

"Allow this sage to cleanse out negative energies and disharmonious entities from this space. All negativity must leave and do no harm so as to allow beneficial energies to bless my home or space." Then focus on the blessings.

Your intention is the main focus in doing this type of cleansing. Your intention is to rid the home of negative

energies and spirits—and they will know this, if they are there. At the same time, the focus is to visualize light and harmony. You can also visualize a geometric shape that looks like an upside-down L with the corner cut on a 90° angle. This is a famous bio-geometry shape that was introduced by Dr. Ibrahim Karim, Egyptian architect, scientist, professor and founder of the Bio-Geometry sciences. (visit www. biogeometry.com) His bio-geometry tools and teachings can be utilized for further clearing and cleansing. Other tools presented by Dr. Robert Gilbert in his work (www.vesica.org) can also be utilized. Always work with your own intuition, drawing a divine power from within your innermost being. There are more techniques and systems that can be of great help that one can learn to do for their homes or offices. Contact the Energy Wellness Institute to learn more about this.

Some people like to re-visit a cleansed house by going back into all of the rooms with pleasant incense such as lavender while inviting all loving, protecting, positive spirits into the home. You may end the ritual by lighting a white candle and setting it on a table to burn for a bit to "seal" your intention.

It is best that the cleansing of the space be done regularly, once a week at least, to do a full smudge for your house. Several times a week would be helpful to smudge your own body and the bodies of the family and friends that live with you.

I like to create a simple "smudge" by adding oils like Sacred Frankincense, Palo Santo or Sage to a spray bottle and spritzing the energy field around myself and the people around me. You can do this for your family and then do the same for each room in your home.

Sacred Frankincense resin can be purchased from Young Living and used in an incense burner for doing this type of space cleansing. This is a great way to air your home and it is helpful to do this or any type of spritzing before your meditation.

ADD MEDITATIONS OR 'QUIET TIME'

The groundbreaking work of Dr. Rick Strassman introduced to the world the role of DMT (which he termed "the Spirit Molecule"). DMT is, as will be discussed in the next chapter, the active agent in a variety of altered states including mystical experiences.

Strassman writes:

> "Meditative techniques using sound, sight, or the mind may generate particular wave patterns whose fields induce resonance in the brain. **Millennia of human trial and error have determined that certain "sacred" words, visual images, and mental exercises exert uniquely desired effects.** Such effects

may occur because of the specific fields they generate within the brain. These fields cause multiple systems to vibrate and pulse at certain frequencies. We can feel our minds and bodies resonate with these spiritual exercises. Of course, the pineal gland also is buzzing at these same frequencies…The pineal begins to "vibrate" at frequencies that weaken its multiple barriers to DMT formation: the pineal cellular shield, enzyme levels, and quantities of anti-DMT. The end result is a psychedelic surge of the pineal spirit molecule, resulting in the subjective states of mystical consciousness."

May you be blessed in your endeavours in achieving, bliss, peace, harmony, happiness—your 'heaven on earth' in your homes!

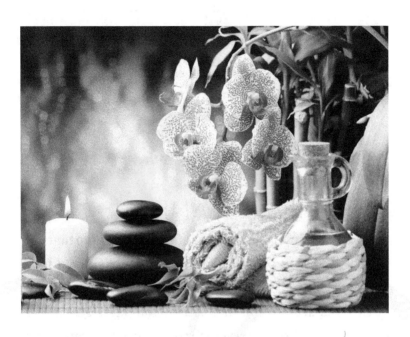

CHAPTER 5:

Green your home & activate your intuitive center: The Pineal Gland

*"The light of the body is the eye:
if therefore thine eye be single, thy
whole body shall be full of light"*

[Matthew 6:22]

CHAPTER 5:

THE "THIRD EYE" OR PINEAL GLAND

The pineal gland is part of one of the most important and least understood systems of our bodies, considered to be the center of our intuition. This organ, the size of a grain of rice, lies deep within the human brain at its geometrical center and has been a mystery for nearly two thousand years.

It is a very active organ, having the **second highest blood flow** after the kidneys and equal in volume to the pituitary. The pineal has the highest absorption of phosphorus in the whole body and the *second highest absorption of iodine,* after the thyroid. No other part of the brain contains so much serotonin or is capable of making melatonin.

The pineal gland is unique in the body: It is an unpaired midline organ in the brain which, alone of all equivalent organs, has resisted encroachment by the corpus callosum. Whilst being right in the centre of the brain, **it is actually outside the blood-brain barrier and so is theoretically not part of the brain!**

Visualizing the third eye

During my years of meditation, through focus and constant discipline in quieting my mind and going within, I also experienced a new vision, a greater perspective of life. **It was as if a light was turned on in my head and I could see and understand life differently.** As I continued to learn various Oriental practices, I became more intrigued with the pineal gland or the third eye chakra.

During a meditation exercise in one of my classes, we were asked to focus on our higher "dantian" center located directly between the eyebrows. **I experienced a most peaceful feeling along, with the vision of a beautiful lotus in full bloom, purplish-indigo in color, located in my brow.** I was surprised later when the instructor informed me that, traditionally among yogis and other Oriental practices, the pineal is known as the thousand-petaled lotus flower. It is symbolized by 1,072 petals, the most petals of any of the energy centres (also referred to as chakras).

Qi Gong and other Oriental schools of thought distinguish three levels of "qi" or energy within the human body: the higher dantian (pineal-brow), middle dantian (heart center) and lower dantian (solar or primal qi). In these teachings, students are often instructed to center their mind in the higher dantian. This is believed to assist in **controlling thoughts and emotions, bringing a deeper sense of calmness, centeredness and peace.**

What is most important is to harmonize our three main energy centers – or the higher, middle and lower Dan-Tian in the body-mind. Dr. Robert Gilbert – author, researcher and lecturer on sacred geometry, Bio-Geometry and sacred initiations addresses this issue in a different and most enlightened way. He teaches the alignment of these three centers: the thinking mind - the brow-3rd eye, to the heart-mind-feeling and then to the navel or Hara centre for grounding and anchoring ourselves. He states how this will maximize our stability in our inner knowing.

When I began taking Kirlian aura photos of my clients with an advanced, scientifically validated Russian instrument called the Gas Discharge Visualization Kirlian camera[1], invented by world renowned physicist Dr. Konstantin Korotkov, I could see areas of energy depletion or disturbances in my clients' bio-fields on a consistent basis. (what is more popularly called the "aura").

I predominantly saw that the brain area in almost all of my clients—from all parts of the world—was showing depletion. Particularly disturbing, was the pineal-pituitary disruption in the brain area. **I observed a direct and severe correlation between pineal-pituitary depletion and continual use of cell phones.**

As I continued to note this and teach about my findings, I began to research the role of the pineal gland even further.

Why is the pineal gland so important?

The first written record of the pineal gland was by Greek physician Herophilus in the third century B.C. Herophilus was an Alexandrian physician who is often called the father of anatomy and the inventor of the scientific method. He was the first to theorize that the spirit of man resided in the pineal center.

Herophilus identified the small pineal structure as being singular, unlike other brain features that are mirrored in the left and right brain hemispheres. He noted that the pineal is the first gland to be formed in the foetus—it is distinguishable at 3 weeks. The pineal gland is also highly nourished, being supplied with the best blood, oxygen and nutrient mix available in the human anatomy, second only to that of our kidneys (whose function is to filter the blood of impurities). Herophilus concluded that this gland had a major role in consciousness and was the gateway to our real self, due to its unique and special anatomical configuration.

Interestingly, it is the only part of the brain that isn't divided into two hemispheres, and is an integral part of the endocrine system. 17th-century French philosopher-mathematician René Descartes regarded it as the **"principal seat of the soul"** and the place in which all our thoughts are formed. He believed that it was **the point of connection, the meeting place of the physical and spiritual, between the intellect and the body.** The body and spirit not only meet there, but each affects the other and the repercussion extends in both directions.

Descartes, like Herophilus, attached great significance to the *pineal gland* because he believed it to be the only section of the brain which existed as a single part rather than one half of a pair.

Obviously, the pineal was considered a very important organ in ancient times: The symbol of the pineal (the pine cone) is found on the staff of the Pope and of the Egyptian god Osiris.

The pineal is considered a portal to the inner or higher self by yogi masters, including Paramahansa Yogananda, author of *Autobiography of a Yogi*. Psychics consider this gland to be the link for interdimensional experiences. It is associated with what many call the third eye or sixth chakra, which is a doorway to higher consciousness and bliss.

In one form of Yoga practice, called Shiva yoga, the primary focus is on awakening the pineal gland. According to the postulates of yoga (specifically those written by H. H. Mahatapaswi Shri Kumarswamiji), **the pituitary gland of the sixth chakra and the pineal gland of the seventh chakra must join their essence in order to open the third eye.** Yogis espouse that this gland is dormant due to our focus on the physical world. When using certain yoga practices, it is possible to activate the connection that merges these glands, resulting in the *'awakening' or activation of this centre.*

In the Bible quote at the top of this chapter, it's significant that the light of the whole body is dependent on the **eye**—the **single eye** that, when full of light, lights the whole body. The pineal has been called the 'Oracle of Light" or the third eye.

In terms of geomagnetic placement, **the pineal gland is the most important part of the body.** It's our magnetic organ. When the pineal gland is vibrant, there is the potential to make rapid leaps in spiritual development and illumination. It is said that the pineal gland is what connects us with the unknowable, the great mystery, the great beyond.

This is our doorway to the creator. If it's blocked, we can't acquire Divine information.

Modern science and philosophy

In recent years, findings in neurochemistry and anthropology have given greater credence to the folklore that **the pineal gland is the 'third eye', source of 'second sight', 'seat of the soul', or psychic centre within the brain.**

The pineal gland synthesizes and secretes melatonin, a structurally simple hormone that communicates information about environmental lighting to various parts of the body, affects the modulation of wake/sleep patterns and reproductive and seasonal functions. The light-transducing ability of the pineal gland equates with the idea that it represents the "third eye".

The biological activity of **melatonin** has also shown it be a potent free radical scavenger, also known as an antioxidant. The precursor to melatonin is serotonin, a neurotransmitter that itself is derived from the amino acid tryptophan. Within the pineal gland, serotonin is acetylated and then methylated to yield melatonin.

Melatonin isn't the only hormone produced in the pineal gland; it also creates a recently discovered substance called **pinoline.** Pinoline is superior to melatonin in aiding DNA replication. It can make superconductive elements within the body. It encourages cell division by resonating with the very pulse of life—at 8 cycles per second, the pulse DNA uses to replicate.

This neurohormone is also thought to be responsible in triggering "dream states", which studies suggest make you more likely to have psychic experiences.

In his book '*DMT, The Spirit* Molecule', Dr. Rick Strassman shows that the pineal gland contains the necessary enzymes and precursors to manufacture di-methyl-tryptamine, or DMT. This is the molecule that he claims is naturally released by the pineal gland, and that facilitates the soul's movement in and out of the body integral in mystical and near death experiences and at the highest states of meditation. **The pineal gland is a source of DMT production during birth, at death and during near-death or mystical experiences. This chemical approach corroborates the idea of the pineal gland as a portal through which the spirit passes through to other dimensions—entering or leaving this physical realm.**

Based on Strassman's groundbreaking research, the film *The Spirit Molecule* weaves an intriguing account of DMT findings. It shows and raises far-reaching theories regarding its role in human consciousness.

Taoist master Mantak Chia considers DMT to be the visual third eye neurotransmitter, produced by the pineal. It enables the energy body and spirit to journey into hyperspace, beyond "third-dimensional realms of time and space." Chia conducts dark room meditations to assist the release of 'endogenous' DMT—in other words, to aid the pineal gland to produce DMT naturally.

According to Chia, **when the pineal gland is activated, it is receiving and converting higher dimensional light into usable information for the pituitary gland.**

Chia speaks of the Crystal Palace, a sacred and spiritually active area deep inside the brain. When the Crystal Palace is activated via darkness and meditation, one can obtain a direct connection with the "source". By focusing on this area of the brain and embracing its darkness, there is the potential for psychic experiences and enlightenment.

Obviously, to have the pineal gland fully activated is an important and much sought after shift for those seeking higher states of consciousness? **A fully activated pineal will assist humanity's spiritual transition from the rule of materialism, greed and enmity to a new period of cooperation, harmony and peace!** When the pineal gland is vibrant, there is the potential to make rapid leaps in spiritual development and illumination. The pineal gland is **Light Made Manifest** in the physical human body.

WHAT BLOCKS THE PINEAL GLAND?

When one's pineal gland becomes blocked or calcified, hormonal production becomes imbalanced. This causes the aging process to accelerate and disrupts the entire Mind-Body-Spirit interplay.

There are many detrimental influences impacting the pineal gland. These include many of the **chemical pollutants used in your cleaning supplies or for your personal hygiene, as well as electromagnetic pollution.** The result of these negative influences is the blocking and hardening (calcification) of your pineal gland.

Remember, the pineal has the highest blood flow per cubic volume than any other organ in the human body! So **whatever is flowing through your blood stream will affect your pineal gland. Let's look at another toxin: fluoride.**

Fluoride

In July 2012, a team of Harvard and Chinese scientists published a study exposing the severe impact of fluoride. Simply, **fluoride lowers IQ**. The report warned of fluoride's potential to reduce human intelligence. The researchers point out that fluoride is a neurotoxicant and issued their warning after reviewing **dozens of studies from the past two decades that have linked elevated fluoride exposure to reduced IQ in children.** Even though the National Research Council issued a similar warning in 2006, advocates of fluoridation continue to push ahead with plans to fluoridate the American people with more water supplies. The United States is the most fluoridated nation on Earth. Fluoridation advocates—including both scientists and city officials—are seriously misrepresenting the data.

"Fluoride seems to fit in with lead, mercury, and other poisons that cause chemical brain drain," senior author of the study Grandjean says. "The effect of each toxicant may seem small, but the combined damage on a population scale can be serious, especially because the brain power of the next generation is crucial to all of us."

What is this doing to our nations in regards to developing **higher awareness**, using **intuitive gifts** and **acquiring direct connection with Source?**

The dangers of fluoride are well-known in producing other side effects. Some of the **known ones in drinking fluoridated water** are dental fluorosis, reduction in childhood intelligence and damage to the nervous system. Fluoride is also known to attack the immune system, an effect confirmed by researchers during a court hearing in Scotland in 1981.* A scientific study, conducted in Belgium, by Oliver, J. (2002,

Aug 11).discovered that excessive use of fluoride products could cause poisoning, damage the nervous system and foster the brittle bone condition, called osteoporosis. http://www.theglobalistreport.com/facts-about-fluoridation-drinking-water

As of December 2012, a total of 42 studies have investigated the relationship between fluoride and human intelligence, and a total of 17 studies have investigated the relationship of fluoride with learning/memory in animals. Of these investigations, 36 of the 42 human studies have found that elevated fluoride exposure is associated with reduced IQ, while 16 of the 17 animal studies have found that fluoride exposure impairs the learning and memory capacity of animals. The human studies, which are based on IQ examinations of over 11,000 children, provide compelling evidence that **fluoride exposure during the early years of life can damage a child's developing brain**.
IQ reductions have been significantly associated with fluoride levels of just 0.88 mg/L among children with iodine deficiency.

Fluoride is particularly harmful, as your body absorbs and **stores fluoride in the pineal gland**. The accumulated fluoride blocks the pineal. Fluoride is a dangerous and toxic substance to the entire body-mind system. It's crucial that you stop using it and drinking it: Avoid fluoridated toothpastes, tooth whiteners or any dental fluoridated tooth cleaning.

To unblock your pineal gland, avoid these things:

- All chemicals and heavy metals— mainly, mercury, fluoride, lead, aluminum and copper. These are toxic to the brain.

- GMO foods

- Pesticides

- Sugar

- Synthetic sweeteners

- Salt

- Acidic beverages (soda pop)

- Beer/wine/alcohol

- Cigarettes (tobacco)

- Pharmaceutical drugs

- Illicit drugs (crack cocaine, cocaine, heroin, etc.)

- Antidepressants

- Marijuana

- Energy drinks

- Negative television programming

- Stress

- Negative emotions, negative or angry people

- Toxic household chemical cleaning products and personal care products

All of these are damaging to the pineal and pituitary glands.

ACTIVATING YOUR PINEAL GLAND

The pineal gland is bioluminescent and sensitive to light. Awakening this gland can speed up our learning, improve our memory ability, enhance our intuition, increase wisdom and creativity, trigger psychic healing abilities and help us experience bliss. Since it is anti-aging, it keeps us vibrant & youthful.

The pineal is vital for supporting intuition, an ability that will be needed during hard times. So it is necessary to evolve spiritually in order to help create better understanding, acceptance of our fellow humans and easier group cooperation.

Meditation is a part of this evolution. Meditation has been known traditionally in many esoteric circles to stimulate this organ, helping you reach higher states of consciousness. **Many meditative practices incorporate sound frequencies to assist in third eye activation** as well as evolving spiritual gifts.

As mentioned earlier, the pineal gland has the highest blood flow of any organ in the human body! Clearly, eating highly nutritious foods that are high in antioxidants will cause healthy nutrients to flow through your blood stream and will positively affect your pineal gland. Sunshine and proper rest can also cause a calcified pineal gland to loosen up, allowing it to open more freely.

As we discussed in Chapter 2, **our sense of smell is our direct route to the pineal** and to the other glands in the brain. Our sense of smell is estimated to be 10,000 times more acute than our other senses, with sensitivity to some 10,000 chemical compounds. There are 800 million nerve endings for processing and detecting odors sending a myriad of messages to the brain instantly. **Through aroma, essential oils have a direct pathway to the pineal gland— which can assist in decalcification and activation.**

Use essential oils to cleanse and stimulate your pineal gland

Chapter 2 had outlined how oil fragrances may be one of the fastest ways to achieve physiological or psychological effects. These same oil fragrances will supercharge your memory and protect your brain from aging and degenerative diseases.

As I considered the major contaminants being used in our homes on a continuous

The best oils to benefit your pineal gland

These Real Green essential oils will help you tremendously to detox and activate the Pineal gland while cleaning, sanitizing, disinfecting or freshening the air in your home or office:

- Brain Power©
- Lemon
- Orange
- Cedarwood
- Vetiver
- Lemongrass
- Sandalwood
- Helichrysum
- Idaho Balsam Fir
- Idaho Blue Spruce
- Inspiration©
- Into the Future©
- Sacred Frankincense

See the Index of Essential Oils for more information!

* Basil

basis and that we could change these products to greener, safer ones, I also realized how much more could be achieved by simultaneously utilizing essential oils for their health impacts to our brains, specifically benefitting the pineal.

Remember, healthy and attuned daily habits will keep your vibrations elevated and your pineal gland stimulated, making you highly intuitive and spiritually enlightened. Create an 'ohm' sound as you inhale the oils to increase vibrational attunement. Once you have completed your cleaning, add extra oil to a diffuser as an air freshener to further enhance and imbue your environment.

The essential oils listed on the side panel (previous page) will help you tremendously to detox and activate the pineal gland while cleaning, freshening, sanitizing or disinfecting your home/office.

A most interesting article that appeared recently addresses this issue of fluoride toxins in our water ways by the use of a well known herbal plant- Tulasi or Holy Basil.

The headlines read, "Researchers discover that the Tulasi Plant Can Be Used To Remove Fluoride from Drinking Water, Providing a Cheap Alternative for the World's Poorest People".

Researchers from Rajasthan University in India have discovered that the **Tulasi plant**, also known as Holy Basil, **can be used to significantly reduce the amount of fluoride in drinking water.**

AN experiment was conducted in the Yellareddyguda village of Narketpally Mandal. The researchers soaked 75mg's of Tulasi leaves in 100ml of water that contained 7.4 parts per million of fluoride in the water.

After only soaking the Tulasi leaves for eight hours, it was discovered that the **level of fluoride in the water was reduced from 7.4 parts per million, to only 1.1 parts per million.**

The significance of this finding is most timely for the removal of a most toxic substance. Basil essential oil will be most useful for many thousands that can also add it to their water as well as use it in the air. As more research is conducted on this, the benefits will be far reaching. http://www.theglobalistreport. com/new-water-treatment-for-removal-of-fluoride/

Here is further information on two powerful essential oils for your pineal gland: with more essential oils described in the Index.

Lemon Essential Oil

Lemon oil, via its vapors alone, will help to cleanse your pineal by digesting the hydrocarbon deposits that block or cloud this gland.

Lemon essential oil promotes clarity of thought and purpose, and has a fragrance that is invigorating, enhancing, and warming. Lemons were used in Europe as early as 200 A.D. and were introduced to the Americas in 1493 by Christopher

Columbus. Lemons were also given to sailors to treat scurvy and other vitamin deficiencies.

Lemon refreshes and stimulates the mind, improves memory and promotes a sense of well-being when diffused. Lemons can be used for basic home remedies. Lemon oil strengthens nails, removes sticky substances and can even be used as an insect repellent when diffused.

In his book The Practice of Aromatherapy, Dr. Jean Valnet M.D. wrote that lemons are a tonic for supporting the nervous and sympathetic nervous system.

Dr. Valnet showed that vaporized lemon oil can kill:

- Menigococcus bacteria in 15 minutes

- Typhoid bacilli in 1 hour

- Staphylococcus aureus in 2 hours

- Pneumococcus bacteria within 3 hours.

Even an 0.2 percent solution of lemon oil can kill diphtheria bacteria in 20 minutes and inactivate tuberculosis bacteria. Lemon oil has been shown to be antitumoral, antiseptic and an immune stimulant (increases white blood cells), and to improve memory. It is rich in natural limonene, a powerful antioxidant, which has been extensively studied for its ability to combat tumor growth in over 50 clinical studies. It is beneficial for obesity, urinary tract infections, varicose veins and digestive problems.

Imagine: while cleaning and disinfecting your home, you're also cleaning or boosting yourself by receiving the immune system benefits of lemon essential oil. This doesn't exist with any other green product. This is truly unique!

See the Index of Essential Oils for the many ways you can use lemon oil in your home or office.

Sacred Frankincense

This is one of the most highly recommended oils for the pineal, due to a new discovery. Sacred Frankincense is a unique and rare type of Frankincense (called Boswellia sacra) from Oman. Omani frankincense is regarded the world over as the rarest, most sought-after aromatic in existence. In Juliet Highet's book *Frankincense: Oman's Gift to the World*, she writes:

> "The international aromatic trade has a grading system for frankincense depending upon size, colour, degree of transparency, and of course fragrance, but it is generally acknowledged that the premium resin comes from Boswellia sacra."

A discovery by Israeli scientist Arieh Moussaieff created headlines around the world when he and an international team of researchers discovered unique capabilities of a constituent in frankincense called Incensole acetate. His studies have shown that **Incensole acetate is in fact responsible for frankincense's remarkable spiritual effects.**

This chemical constituent triggered an ion channel in the brain with heretofore unknown effects. The areas of the brain affected are known to be involved in emotions. Incensole acetate had an anti-anxiety effect and significantly improved mood in the study.

Sacred Frankincense is ideal for those who wish to take their spiritual journey and meditation experiences to a higher level. It also has many other properties, and is used to cleanse and disinfect homes in the Middle East as well as to ward off insects and enhance the immune system.

Becoming spiritually connected will assist in embracing one's true purpose in the world, shift consciousness, awaken to one's higher powers, intuition and become more spiritually driven rather than ego driven.

Frankincense with Lavender or Frankincense with Peppermint is an awesome combination for the diffuser or as an air freshener that stimulates the brain. Can also be applied topically over the forehead.

MORE WAYS TO INCREASE PINEAL ACTIVITY

- Humming while you clean with these oils will further stimulate the brain and pineal center.

- Listen to relaxing music to calm your mind.

- The sound "OM" resonates with the Fourth Chakra, known as the Heart Center, the seat of Unconditional Love. Chanting can be done anytime, anywhere; Chanting "ohm" opens you up to universal and cosmic awareness. You can chant for 5 minutes, 10 minutes, or however long you desire to.

- Diffuse the oils of your choice, close your eyes, relax and meditate. Focus on the forehead, visualize and chant, even if it's only for 10 minutes. Then focus on your heart center, and lastly focus beneath your navel feeling the grounding energy. A few minutes every day can make a huge shift- as it's the repetitiveness and consistency that will impact the most.

- Increase antioxidant foods and herbs in your diet: Chlorella, spirulina and other blue-green algae, iodine, zeolite, ginseng, D3, bentonite clay, chlorophyll, gotu kola, parsley, alfalfa, raw cacao, NIngxia berries, cilantro, watermelon, **Basil**, bananas, honey, coconut oil, hemp seeds, seaweed, ningxia red juice, etc.

Pollution of an unusual sort emanates from electromagnetic sources. This chapter is intended to raise awareness of this modern-day pollutant that is also one of the least understood or identified for many homeowners—and that very much affects the 'greening' of your home.

In order to have safe, vibrant and comfortable homes, homeowners need to address this issue.

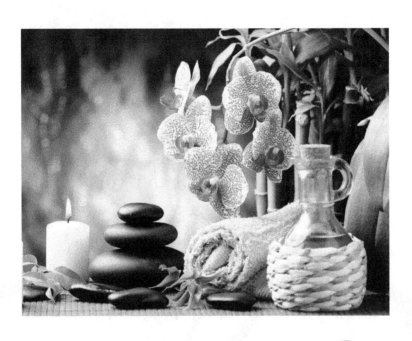

CHAPTER *6*:

Is electromagnetic pollution making you ill?

"Unless it heated tissue, electromagnetic radiation was thought to be harmless. So there were no limits placed on exposure to frequencies below microwave."

– Robert O Becker in Cross Currents

CHAPTER 6:

WHAT IS ELECTROMAGNETIC POLLUTION?

The technologies we use today—from our everyday appliances to cell phones and even our cars—emit electromagnetic radiation that can penetrate and affect us, seriously compromising our health and disturbing our environments.

For years, scientists have conducted research linking EM radiation to serious diseases like cancer, Alzheimer's disease, Parkinson's disease and others.

Research now links long-term exposure to electromagnetic fields (EMFs) with chronic health issues, from stress and fatigue to cancer. Overwhelming numbers of scientists now agree that EMFs are carcinogens. **But like any massive public health threat, it may be years before the talk stops and the action starts. In the meantime, people are getting sick.**

EMFs are created by the spewing forth of our modern day life: cell phones, power lines and other technologies all emit electromagnetic waves. We are exposed to 200,000,000 times more EM fields in our environment today than our ancestors were. This is more than our circuits can handle. EMFs (also called Electro-Smog) are invisible, silent and ubiquitous.

SCIENTIFIC RESEARCH ON EMFS

There are more studies showing the adverse effects of EMFs than there are studies showing risks for cancer by smokers. Here are a few notable reports:

- **EMF is classified as a Group 2B carcinogen** under standards established by the World Health Organization's International Agency for Research on Cancer. The chemicals DDT and lead are also Group 2B carcinogens.

- After an analysis of seven studies, the National Institute of Environmental Health Sciences concluded that EMFS "should be regarded as possible carcinogens."

- An international group of leading researchers recently came out stating, "**the existing standards for public safety are inadequate to protect public health.**"

- In 1989, Dr. Stephen Perry of Britain's National Health Service observed that patients living near power lines had a high incidence of mental problems and a high suicide rate. A follow-up study by Dr. Charles Poole found 2.8 times more depression symptoms in people living near overhead transmission lines.

- Dr. N. Wertheimer, University of Colorado and physicist Edward Leeper found 60 Hertz magnetic fields of only 3 mG were significantly related to a threefold increase in childhood cancers, especially leukemia and brain tumors.

No longer an invisible danger

Researchers and media worldwide are constantly publishing findings on cell phone radiation and its effects on the human body.   People are becoming more informed about 'the damage to your brain cells'.

In 2011, **the World Health Organization "rang alarm bells around the world" when it placed microwave radiation from wireless internet and cell phones on an official cancer watchlist.**

In June 2012, a Toronto hospital was the first to formally recognize symptoms from wireless radiation. Women's College Hospital urged family doctors to learn to detect the symptoms of wireless radiation exposure. They include **disrupted sleep, headaches, nausea, dizziness, heart palpitations, memory problems and skin rashes. This condition is being labelled Electro-magnetic Hyper-sensitivity, or "EMS".**

In July 2012, the American Academy of Pediatrics sponsored legislation that would urge the Federal Communications Commission to strengthen cell phone testing. **The AAP**

states that children are especially vulnerable to damage from cell phone radiation, and should not use cell phones without a headset. This statement is based on the findings of an expert panel on the IARC, which ruled that there was some evidence that regular cell phone use increased the risk of two types of tumors – brain tumors (gliomas) and acoustic neuromas.

> *"Vast numbers of people are using mobile phones and they could be a time bomb of health problems—not just brain tumors, but also fertility, which would be a serious public health issue.*
>
> *"The health effects of smoking, alcohol and air pollution are well known and well talked about, and it's entirely reasonable we should be openly discussing the evidence for this, but it is not happening.*
>
> *"We want to close the door before the horse has bolted."*

- Professor Dennis Henshaw

Children under 16 should minimise their use of mobile phones—and, while using a mobile device, keep your phone at least 15mm away from your bodies at all times. This may come as a surprise to those who keep their phones in their pockets.

We do live in electro-magnetic smog, and people are exposed to wireless devices all the time. Our bodies are being completely bombarded on a continuous basis—from smart meters attached to the homes, cell phones, smart phones and computers and so on. We are now seeing the biological impact and medical researchers and scientists are increasingly stepping forward to share a growing concern.

LEADERS IN EMF RESEARCH

Magda Havas: The Need for Stronger Standards

Dr. Magda Havas is an Associate Professor of Environmental & Resource Studies at Trent University, where she teaches and does research on the biological effects of environmental contaminants. Since the 1990s, she has been quite active and concerned with the biological effects of electromagnetic pollution on human populations, including radio frequency radiation, electromagnetic fields, dirty electricity and ground current. She has been instrumental in raising a greater awareness about the dangers of the EMF pollutant amongst the general population and government bodies. Simply stated, **she advises greater controls in EMF exposures.**

Dr. Havas works with diabetics as well as with individuals who have **multiple sclerosis, tinnitus, chronic fatigue, fibromyalgia** and those who are **electrically hypersensitive**. Havas also conducts research on **sick building syndrome** as it relates to power quality in schools and has become a master in disseminating her findings about EMFs' ill effects.

In 2010, Dr. Havas published a research paper documenting definitive evidence that **radiation from a cordless phone causes heart arrhythmia and tachycardia (rapid heart rate) and alters the sympathetic and parasympathetic nervous system similar to a "fight-or-flight" stress response.**

This study is **the first one of its kind to demonstrate such a dramatic and repeatable response to pulsed-microwave radiation at levels 0.5 percent of federal guidelines in both Canada and the U.S.** The double-blind, peer-reviewed study in the European Journal of Oncology clearly shows that some individuals are hypersensitive to this radiation and react immediately and not only during active provocation.

Dr. Havas' work has revealed a major shortcoming in health standards for radiation in Canada. In fact, we now know that the Safety Code 6 guideline set by Health Canada for microwave radiation (which includes radiation from most of the devices we are concerned about like mobile phones, cell phone antennas, Wi-Fi, wireless toys and baby monitors, smart meters etc.) is based ONLY on preventing a heating effect!

In other words, Health Canada's safety code is *only* concerned with whether electromagnetic radiation between 100 kHz and 300 kHz creates heat—even though radiation at that level is proven to be harmful even without raising your body's temperature!

This is shocking: Health Canada has stated that Safety Code 6 takes into consideration and protects the public from both thermal and non-thermal effects. This statement was in response to groups concerned about Wi-Fi in schools, and to those concerned about smart meters and cell towers coming into their neighborhoods.

Health Canada has misled the public by failing to mention in that the "non-thermal" effects are considered ONLY for frequencies between 3 and 100 kHz. For frequencies between 100 kHz and 300 GHz ONLY thermal effects are considered and cell towers fall within this "thermal range."

Dr. Havas continually educates the general public about the environmental issues of EMFs. She recently wrote, with Camilla Rees, *Public Health SOS: The Shadow Side of the Wireless Revolution*. She has co-edited three books and published more than 100 articles on the subject.

She has been an advisor to several public interest groups, government lobby groups and educational groups concerned with the health of the environment. She is currently science advisor on EMF-related issues to several non-profit organizations.

Devra Davis: The Cell Phone Hush-Up

Dr. Devra Davis is one of the most well-respected and credentialed researchers on the dangers of cell phones. She is founder and president of the Environmental Health

Trust, and acted as the founding director at the U.S. National Academy of Sciences, serving on the Board of Environmental Studies and Toxicology.

Dr. Davis warns that **cell phone radiation is as dangerous as carcinogenic pesticides—which have been banned worldwide**—yet, even though cell phones are classified by the International Agency for Research on Cancer as a Class 2B carcinogen, they are still in common use.

Dr. Davis strongly advises that **you should not keep a cell phone in your pocket or on your body**, and should use an air-tube headset or the speakerphone feature as much as possible, reminding people that 'distance is your friend'.

Dr. Davis shares information about the risks of cell phone use via informational videos, including a recent interview by Dr. Joseph Mercola. (http://youtu.be/rnhSwiL0QAg)

In the interview, Dr. Davis points out that **a cell phone is a two-way microwave-radiating device** that has been associated with brain tumors and salivary gland tumors; weakened sperm production, vitality and quantity; hearing loss and tinnitus; and many other health issues.

She reports that an Israeli research group is warning of **a sharp increase in the incidence of parotid gland tumors over the last 30 years, with the steepest increase happening after 2001.** Your parotid gland is a type of salivary gland, located closest to your cheek—the same area where most people typically hold their cell phones. The researchers found a four-fold increase in parotid gland cancers from 1970 to 2006, while rates of other salivary gland cancers remained stable.

Dr. Davis says: "In Israel, one in five cases now is under the age of 20. **This is a very rare tumor, but it is occurring in young people.** That is why the Israeli government has issued warnings about children using cell phones. The Israeli Dental Association has issued a warning as well, because of the dramatic increase in a very rare and malignant tumor of the cheek."

She also points out that **the telecommunications industry is a global multi-trillion dollar industry that influences government policies through persistent lobbying efforts, sizeable political donations and manipulation of science. Is our government truly protecting us from the dangers of cell phone radiation?**

George Carlo: A tumor epidemic

As a matter of fact, **many scientists were warned not to reveal their findings.** This was the case with Dr. George Carlo. Dr. Carlo is a medical researcher and epidemiologist who headed the first telecommunications industry-backed studies into the dangers of cell phone use, from 1993 to 1999. **His $28.5 million research program was funded by the cell phone industry to prove the safety of wireless technology,**

but ended up doing exactly the opposite: Dr. Carlo proved that cell phones are dangerous!

Confirmed by major studies worldwide, Dr. Carlo's work convinced the insurance industry to cancel product liability coverage for EMF radiation injury cases from cell phones. **Dr. Carlo predicted a potential epidemic by 2010, reaching 500,000 new tumor cases every year.** He states that teenagers and children are especially vulnerable. As he predicted, tumor cases amongst children have escalated.

EMFS AND YOUR PINEAL GLAND

There are other researchers who have been specifically studying the pineal gland with EMF's. In my own work with the GDV Kirlian camera, I consistently noticed bio-field changes--sometimes huge gaps would appear above and around the head area, which (as explained in Chapter 5) became my alarm bell.

In one study, Malka N. Halgamuge investigated pineal melatonin level disruption from EMF exposures. The author observed that **with the high daily usage of electricity, exposure to power-frequency (50 or 60 Hz) EMFs is unavoidable. So what is the impact on the brain?** Melatonin, as discussed in Chapter 5, is a natural hormone produced by pineal gland activity in the brain that regulates the body's sleep–wake cycle. In this study, more than one hundred experimental data of human and animal studies of changes in melatonin levels due to power-frequency electric and magnetic fields exposure were analyzed.

The results showed the significance of disruption of melatonin due to exposure to weak EMFs, which the author states, **may possibly lead to long-term health effects in humans.**

Another study examined the possible effects of 60-Hz electromagnetic field exposure on pineal gland function in humans. In the study, the researchers measured excretion of urinary 6-hydroxymelatonin sulfate (6-OHMS), a stable urinary metabolite of the pineal hormone melatonin, in 42 individuals who used conventional and continuous polymer wire (CPW) electric blankets for the duration of 8 weeks.

Their findings were significant enough that the researchers hypothesized that **exposure to extremely low frequency electric or magnetic fields can affect pineal gland function.**

A third study was conducted at the University of Berne in Switzerland. The researchers wanted to ascertain the effects of 16.7 Hz magnetic fields on 6-hydroxymelatonin sulfate or 6-OHMS excretion. This study compared 6-OHMS levels of 108 male railway workers between leisure periods and days following the start of service on electrically powered engines or working beneath transmission lines. The findings were similar:

"The results support the hypothesis that 16.7 Hz magnetic fields alter 6-OHMS excretion in humans."

More solutions are coming forth for neutralizing these radiation exposures.

WHAT YOU NEED TO KNOW ABOUT EMFS

The amount of environmental toxins that all of us contend with has reached unprecedented levels. By being aware of these pollutants, you can take action—not just by limiting your household chemical usage, but by limiting your exposure to the electromagnetic soup we stew in.

As we have seen, **human consciousness is affected by the performance of the pineal gland**, and as it has been demonstrated, the pineal gland is adversely affected by environmental electro-magnetic radiation and by chemical toxins. **We are damaging our consciousness with over-exposures from all of these poisons.**

By changing our ways, we will ensure that our brains and pineal glands are protected, so that we may elevate our consciousness, journey into the higher planes and gain wisdom and illumination, all while increasing our intuitive abilities.

Visit electromagneticpollution.weebly.com for more information and upcoming solutions to balancing EMF exposures.

Solutions will be posted as to what you can do to transmute harmful EMF's.

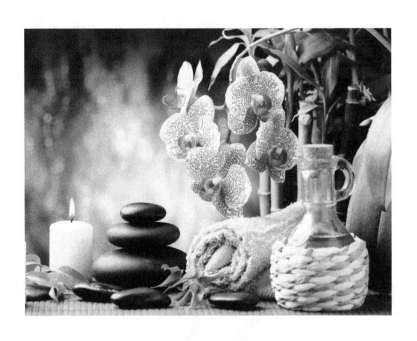

CHAPTER 7:

Your eco-green guide to Vibrational Cleaning

Use common 'scents' to go green, energetically attune your home or office and activate your pineal gland!

CHAPTER 7:

Now you know how important it is to use safe, natural and truly beneficial cleaning supplies in your home or office. I have created this **Real Green Essentials©- Vibrational** guide for you, so you can reap the cleaning power, energy benefits and therapeutic joy from the use of Nature's purest elements: essential oils.

KITCHEN

Scouring Powder
- To one cup of baking soda, add 20 drops of Lemon, Purification, Lavender, Cypress, Orange, Palmarosa or Lemongrass oil. Mix well to infuse the powder. Apply on a damp sponge and use as your surface cleaner, enjoying the aromas as you clean.

Dishes
- For sparkling dishes, add 1 to 2 tablespoons of Thieves Household Cleaner, along with 2 to 3 drops of Lemon, Orange or Melrose oil. It will

create a great smelling kitchen by diffusing the oils. Beneficial to inhale.

- Make dishwasher detergent by adding 3 to 4 drops of Lemon, Citrus Fresh, Melrose or Orange oil to washing soda.

Oven Cleaner

- Clean your oven soon after a spill with moistened baking soda and 3 drops of Lavender, Lemon, Lemongrass or Tangerine oil. Let stand until softened and wipe clean.

Refrigerator

- To clean your refrigerator, spray Thieves Household Cleaner on the doors and shelves, and wipe with a damp cloth. You can also clean shelves and drawers with Thieves wipes.

- To fight odors, add one drop of Grapefruit, Orange, Bergamot, or Lemon to a wet cloth, then wipe the shelves. Deodorizes and prevents odours from penetrating other foods.

Rubbish Bins

- Clean, deodorize and disinfect with hot water and 3 to 4 drops of any of these oils: Eucalyptus, Melaleuca, Melrose, or Oregano.

- Deodorize by adding one drop of the above oils into the bin every now and then (at least twice weekly).

Water Purification

- To a gallon of water, add 1 to 2 drops of Peppermint, Oregano, Mountain Savoury, Thieves or Cinnamon oil.

Stainless Steel Cleaner

- Remove smudges/marks from stainless steel appliances with 3 drops of Lemon or Purification oil, added to one tablespoon of olive oil. Mix well. Dip a rag into the oil mixture and rub the surface to rid smudges. Apply vinegar onto another rag – wipe and let dry.

Food Preparation

Yes, you can use these same essential oils to keep your food safe, healthy and flavorful!

- Add 1 or 2 drops to your recipes towards the end of cooking or your food preparations. This will help to keep the flavor strong. Add as per your favourite taste and recipe: Lemon, Lime, Lavender, Rosemary, Marjoram, Oregano, Peppermint, and Orange or Tangerine oil.

For example:

- Season salad dressings with lemon, oregano, rosemary or peppermint.

- Season baked goods (frostings, puddings, fruit pies) with lemon, lime, tangerine or lavender.

- Marinade with an added drop of oils: create a mixture for your vegetables, fruit, or any meat/ fish

- Add to hot water for your favorite herbal tea: peppermint, lemon, or lavender

- Flavour honey or agave with your choice of oil including raw cacao. Delicious!

Dual-purpose food spray

As discussed earlier, **oregano and thyme** oil can disinfect your cutting board, preserve your food and add flavor.

- Simply fill a spray bottle half full with filtered water; add **20 drops of oregano, thyme, marjoram and/ or cinnamon oil;** shake and spritz where needed.

Remember, since these oils are GRAS approved as food enhancers, they can be used on your food as well as your disinfecting cleansing agents.

Soaking Fruits and Vegetables

Add a few drops of essential oils of **Lemon, Thieves, Lime, Orange or Purification** to a sink filled with cold water- with 2 tablespoons of **Thieves household cleaner**.

Soak your fruits and vegetables for a few minutes as this will help to wash off parasites, pesticides and other bacteria. It also breaks down wax or other coatings added by growers and helps fruits and vegetables store longer.

BATHROOM

All-purpose cleaning spray

- For tiles, countertops, floors, tubs. To one gallon of hot water, add ½ cup of white vinegar, 1 tablespoon of Borax, and 15 drops of **Lemongrass, Oregano, Lemon or Palmarosa oil**.

General bathroom cleaner

- Use any of the following oils as a room spray or surface cleaner: **Oregano, Orange, Bergamot, Lemon, Lemongrass, Palmarosa or Lavender.** Put 2 to 3 drops directly on a wet wash cloth, or use 8 drops in 2 litres of washing water.

- Use Oregano on a wash cloth to disinfect countertops and sinks.

Disinfectant

- Mix 50 to 100 drops of **Eucalyptus oil** with a litre of water. Shake and use in a spray bottle. Eucalyptus oil is a good disinfectant and deodorizer. It gets rid of some stains like ink and grease, kills and repels some insects. *It'll even attack rust.*

- Disinfect wash cloths by soaking them in a bowl of boiling water with a few drops of Eucalyptus, Lavender, Purification, Melaleuca, Thyme,

Oregano, or Citrus Fresh oil before washing.

- Disinfectant blend: To a small bowl of water, add 2 drops of Lavender oil, 4 drops of Thyme oil, 1 drop of Eucalyptus oil and 1 drop of Oregano oil.

- Lemon, Spruce, or Fir oil can also be used for disinfecting bathrooms and kitchens.

- Soak toothbrushes in solution of Oregano oil, Thieves oil, Melrose oil or Melaleuca oil in salted water to combat microbes. Add a couple of drops to your toothbrush with Thieves toothpaste.

Toilets

- Use Oregano oil for disinfecting toilets. Add a few drops every day.

- Use 2 to 3 drops of Lemon, Citrus Fresh, Palmarosa or Eucalyptus oil for cleaning. Scrub toilet and let stand a few minutes.

Air freshening

- Use 2 drops of Purification, Rosemary, Melaleuca, Eucalyptus or Grapefruit oil on the cardboard inner ring of toilet roll.

- Create your own natural potpourri with dried flowers and add oils.

- For a deodorizing spray, mix **2 drops Rosemary, 4 drops Lemon, 3 drops Eucalyptus and 4 drops Lavender** in 1 quart of water. Shake well.

LAUNDRY

- Add 2 or 3 drops of lemon oil to water and spray the laundry room, counter tops and sinks as lemon oil will help sanitize them.

- Use other oils like Thieves, Palmarosa, Lavender or Melrose

- Wipe the countertops and sinks with the Thieves handi-wipes - available from Young Living company.

Washing

Add essential oils to your laundry to increase anti-bacterial benefits and to provide greater hygiene.

- Use Thieves Household Cleaner in your wash water.

- Recent research has shown that ***Eucalyptus oil kills dust mites***. Dust mites live in your bedding, feeding from the dead skin cells you constantly shed. To kill dust mites, **add 25 drops of Eucalyptus oil to each wash load.**

- As a softening agent, add a dampened wash cloth loaded with 10 drops of Lavender, Lemon, or Melaleuca oil.

- Add a couple of drops of Lemon, Lavender, Rosemary, Purification, Lemongrass, Citrus Fresh or Bergamot oil to the final rinse water.

- Add 2 to 3 drops of Lavender, Joy, Palmarosa, or Bergamot oil directly to the clothes in your dryer, or on a small cloth.

- Soak your dishcloth or other laundry items overnight in a bowl of water with one drop of lemon oil to help to sanitize them.

- Use a drop or two of lemon essential oil on stains. Let stand, and rub off with a clean cloth or throw into laundry cycle. Lemon oil can also help remove gum, oil, grease spots or crayon.

Drying

- Add Thieves wipes to your dryer.

- Instead of using toxic and irritating softening sheets in the dryer, toss in a dampened washcloth with 10 **drops of lavender, lemon, melaleuca, bergamot**, or other oils added. While the oils will not reduce static cling, they will impart a lovely, clean, refreshing fragrance to your clothes.

- To prevent static cling- simply roll aluminum foil into a ball and add to your dryer.

GENERAL CLEANING

Disinfect with Thieves Wipes

- Thieves Wipes are ideal for use on door handles, toilet seats and any surface that needs cleaning to protect from dust, mold, and undesirable microorganisms. Keep a pack handy in your bathroom, laundry room, kitchen, car, office, or anywhere else you want to keep your environment clean without toxic chemicals. Thieves essential oil blend has been university tested for its effects against unwanted microorganisms and found to be highly effective in supporting the immune system and good health. (See Chapter 3)

Furniture Polish

- In a spray bottle, combine ½ cup of vegetable oil with 2 tablespoons of white or cleaning vinegar and 10 to 15 drops of **Spruce, Cedarwood, Cypress, Fir, Lemon, Vetiver or Lavender** oil. Shake, spray and polish with a rag. Test on the wood beforehand.

Mirrors, Glass, Windows

- Make a cleaning spray with equal parts vinegar and water, and **10 drops of Lemon, Lime or Grapefruit oil**. Use a paper or microfiber towel.

- After washing, add one drop of **Lemon, Lime or Grapefruit** oil to a newspaper or paper towel and rub over windows to remove streaky marks.

Closets

- Make your linens smell fresh by adding oil to the cupboard liner or strips of blotting paper: **Lavender, Chamomile, Marjoram, Rosemary or Palmarosa**.

- For fresh and moth-free clothes, spray a few drops of **Lavender** or **Eucalyptus** into the closets and drawers.

- Make a sachet by placing several drops of

Citronella, Lavender, Lemongrass or Rosemary oil on a cotton ball. Wrap and tie it into a small handkerchief. Hang in storage areas.

- Deodorize smelly shoes: Add oil to strips of blotting paper and place in shoes overnight. Use 2 to 3 drops of **Eucalyptus, Lemongrass, Bergamot, Cypress, Lavender, or Purification**. The oils can also be applied directly into the shoes.

Floors and Carpets

- Hardwood floors: Add ¼ cup white vinegar to a bucket of water. Add 5 to 10 drops of **Lemon, Cedarwood or Fir** oil. OR *Brain Power, Inspiration or Into The Future*

- Carpet freshener: Add 16 to 20 drops of **Lemon, Citrus Fresh, Lavender or Bergamot oil** to a cup of baking soda. Mix well and cover overnight. Then sprinkle it over your carpet, wait 10 minutes and vacuum.

Special Deodorizing Spray

This spray deodorizes and cleans the air instead of masking the odors—a real odor eater!

Ingredients:

- 2 drops rosemary essential oil

- 4 drops lemon essential oil

- 2 drops eucalyptus (E. globulus) essential oil

- 4 drops lavender essential oil

- 1 quart distilled water or purified water

- Fill a 1 quart spray bottle with water, add the essential oils and mix by shaking the bottle. Use to clean the air or even on countertops, sinks, tiles or cupboards.

Hot tubs and saunas:

- Use 3 drops per person of **lavender, cinnamon, clove, eucalyptus, thyme, lemon,** or grapefruit essential oil to disinfect and freshen the water. Can add **Brain Power, Sacred Frankincense or Inspiration**

- For saunas, add several drops of **rosemary, thyme, pine, or lavender** oil to a spray bottle with water, and spray surfaces. This water can also be used to splash onto hot sauna stones.

AIR FRESHENING

You can use any essential oil as an air freshener to gain its therapeutic benefits. See the Index of Essential Oils to learn more, or use one of my favorites:

- **Lavender**: improves sleep quality and calms the nervous system

- **Idaho Balsam Fir:** helps relieve headaches, stress, sore muscles and tension

- **Peppermint:** stimulates the mind and improves memory

- **Thieves oil**: helps relieve nasal congestion, stuffiness

- **Lemon**: acts as a natural antidepressant and calms anxiety

- **Orange**: refreshes and relaxes

- Basic air freshener: Simply add distilled water with 10-20 drops of your favorite oil and spray in any room. The spritzer can also be used for spraying your linens, bedding and towels.

- Use a cold-air oil diffuser. This is a great way to infuse your home with a continuous and subtle scent. Use Brain Power, Inspiration or Idaho Balsam Fir to especially activate the pineal, or choose Lemon, Lime or any of the citrus oils to help decalcify.

- Create your own potpourri: Use a crystal vase, china dish or wicker basket and add dried flower petals, pinecones or lavender florets. Then simply sprinkle your essential oil over it. Choose your oil according to what room you'd like to use this in. (see my Eco Green Your Holidays video on Rogers TV: http://www.rogerstv.com/page.aspx?lid=237&rid=51&gid=105025)

- Use rice as a potpourri: Fill a small decorative jar or dish with plain white rice and add in a few drops of oil. Place the jar in whatever room you wish to fill with the fragrance. I use peppermint or lemon for the bathroom and lavender for the bedroom.

- Create a hanging sachet with your essential oil of choice for activating the pineal. This is especially helpful in your office and bedroom. Add dried florets or pine cones to a mesh bag; add drops of your favorite pineal-stimulating essential oils.

- Infuse blotting paper or a clay pendant to hang in closets, laundry room and or bathrooms.

- Apply a few drops of lavender, or another calming essential oil, onto a cotton ball for your pillows. Place the cotton inside your pillowcase to help calm your senses as you drift off to sleep. Better still, add drops of one of the pineal activation oils- **Brain Power, Into The Future, or Inspiration or Blue Spruce**

- Dab cotton balls with essential oils and place in the corners of your drawers and closets. This tip not only helps with keeping clothes smelling fresh, but it also helps ward off moths!

Added tip: Use houseplants to detoxify and improve your air quality. A number of plants have been studied for their healthy air benefits. The *spider plant*, for example, was researched by NASA and found that it can reduce dangerous levels of toxins in a room by *96 percent in 24 hours.*

STEPS TO ELIMINATING MOLD

As discussed in Chapter 3, mold can produce a variety of unhappy and even dangerous ailments. To eradicate and protect yourself from toxic mold, follow this regimen.

Remember: This is for What you can do? At Home Mold Cleaning

What to Wear When Cleaning Moldy Areas

It is important to take precautions to **LIMIT YOUR EXPOSURE** to mold and mold spores.

1) Find if there is a leak or if there is a humidity problem first so that you can call in the experts to rectify this problem

2) **Use a mask:** In order to limit your exposure to airborne mold, you may want to wear an **N-95 respirator** (as recommended by the EPA). It is important to avoid breathing **in mold or mold spores.** The respirator is available at many hardware stores and from companies that advertise on the Internet (They cost about $12 to $25.) The respirator or mask must fit properly to be effective, so carefully follow the instructions supplied with the respirator.

3) **Wear gloves:** Long gloves that extend to the middle of the forearm are recommended. When working with water and a mild detergent, ordinary household rubber gloves may be used. Avoid touching mold or moldy items with your bare hands.

4) **Wear goggles:** EPA recommends Goggles that do not have ventilation holes as a way to protect your eyes. Avoid getting mold or mold spores into your eyes.

Other Tips:

- **Fix plumbing leaks and other water problems as soon as possible. Dry all items completely.**

- **Follow the 'Thieves Mold Removal' listed below before you begin the Mold cleanup.**

- Absorbent or porous materials, such as ceiling tiles and carpet, clothing or furnishings may need to be thrown away if they become moldy. Make sure that these items are placed and sealed in an airtight plastic bag.

- Avoid exposing yourself or others to mold

- Do not paint or caulk moldy surfaces. Clean up the mold first and dry the surfaces before painting. Paint applied over moldy surfaces is likely to peel.

- If you are unsure about how to clean an item, or if the item is expensive or of sentimental value, you may wish to consult a specialist.

- Increase ventilation in closed areas such as bathrooms- (running a fan or opening a window) and cleaning more frequently will usually prevent mold from recurring, or at least keep the mold to a minimum.

Overview

Dr. Edward Close, whose work in eliminating mold with the use of Thieves essential oils was discussed in Chapter 3, highly recommends the method detailed below.

To diffuse Thieves essential oil, use a waterless or cold air diffuser, in the infested area and throughout the house. One 15ml bottle of Thieves will cover 1,000 square feet. You can run several diffusers at once.

The more that the area is saturated with the aromatic compounds, the more effective the procedure will be. It is also important to use Thieves Household Cleaner to clean all areas, floor, ceilings, walls, bedding, countertops, etc. after diffusing.

Materials

- Thieves essential oil
- cold-air diffuser
- pail, mop and sponge
- rubber gloves

Basic Non-Toxic Mold Removal

1) Sample first to determine the type of mold (toxic or non-toxic) that is present.

2) After samples have been collected, diffuse the Thieves Essential Oil Blend for 24 to 72 hours, non-stop in the space(s) where mold was found. Leave the room closed and sealed during this intensive diffusing.

3) Contact a professional to repair all leaks and eliminate all sources of moisture into the premises.

4) NO toxic mold after diffusing – clean visible mold with undiluted Thieves Household Cleaner, with gloves and mask.

5) Remove & seal any mold-infested materials in plastic & throw them away.

6) If toxic mold was found, then contact a professional for mold assistance.

- protective mask- **N-95 respirator**
- Thieves Household Cleaner

Mold prevention

As a preventative, diffuse Thieves Essential Oil Blend for 8 hours continuously every week in your environment, or diffuse for 15 minutes every 3 hours. You'll be glad that you have.

THIEVES MOLD REMOVAL - STEPS

Eliminate mold and prevent it from returning!
CAUTION: If your home or space is saturated with mold, then contact a professional.

1) Sample first to determine the type of mold present (toxic or non-toxic). Toxic mold must be dealt with differently than non-toxic mold.

2) After samples have been collected, diffuse the Thieves Essential Oil Blend for 24 to 72 hours, non-stop, in the space(s) where mold was found. A cold-air diffuser, available via Young Living, works well in spaces up to 1000 sq. ft. in size. For best results, leave the room closed and sealed during this intensive diffusing. This will allow maximum penetration and absorption of the essential oil blend to inactivate the mold spores.

3) Contact a professional to repair all leaks and eliminate all sources of moisture into the premises.

4) If NO toxic mold was found, then after diffusing has been completed, clean visible mold with undiluted Thieves Household Cleaner. Use gloves, masks and other protective equipment. It is important to take precautions to avoid touching and breathing mold spores while cleaning.

5) Remove any mold-infested materials, seal them in plastic and throw them away.

6) If toxic mold was found, then contact a professional mold remediation service to have infested materials removed and to have them properly disposed of as these are hazardous materials. Diffuse in the sealed off space for 24 to 72 hours non-stop. Repairs must be done and infested materials replaced.

7) Have your professional resample to be sure all sources of mold have been identified and remediated. Repair all affected areas

8) If necessary, repeat the above steps 1 through 6, above.

9) Diffuse regularly for prevention and protection on a weekly basis or short periods each day.

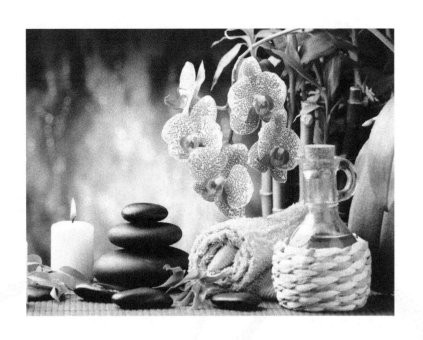

CHAPTER *8*:

Go real green with really natural deodorants!

Use common 'scents' under your arms

CHAPTER 8:

HOW TOXIC ARE YOUR DEODORANTS/ ANTIPERSPIRANTS?

Did you know? Scientists in Britain suggest they may have found **a possible link between the use of deodorants and breast cancer.**

Back in 2007, scientists measured aluminum content in breast tissue from breast cancer patients and found that the aluminum content of breast tissue was higher in the region where there would be the highest density of antiperspirant. Aluminum chloride—the active ingredient in antiperspirants—has been found to act similarly to the way oncogenes work, facilitating molecular transformations in cancer cells. Aluminum salts also mimic estrogen, and bio-accumulate in breast tissue, which can raise your breast cancer risk.

Other major toxins included:

- **Propylene Glycol** – used in anti-freeze, this chemical is implicated in contact dermatitis, kidney damage and liver abnormalities; can inhibit skin cell growth in human tests and can damage cell membranes causing rashes, dry skin and surface damage.

- **Triclosan** – Used as an antibacterial agent, this chemical has endocrine-disrupting properties amongst many other toxic effects. (See Chapter 1)

- **Parabens** – Known to have an estrogen-mimicking effect. Estrogen is well-known to play a key role in the development, growth and progression of breast cancer. (See Chapter 1)

Recent research found also higher concentrations of parabens in the upper quadrants of the breast and axillary area, where antiperspirants are usually applied, suggesting they too may contribute to the development of breast cancer.

In one shocking study, researchers at the University of Reading in the UK studied tissue samples taken from 40 women who had undergone mastectomies for breast cancer, and found that **99 percent of all tissue samples contained at least one paraben.** Worse, 60 percent of the samples contained five parabens.

Overall, topical applications of personal care products that contain parabens appear to be the greatest source of exposure to these estrogen-mimicking chemicals, far surpassing the risk of the aluminum in antiperspirants.

DEODORANT AND ANTIPERSPIRANT FACTS

- Sweat has no odor; the familiar unpleasant odor is caused by bacteria that live on our skin and hair. These bacteria metabolize the proteins and fatty acids from our apocrine sweat, causing body odor.

- Deodorants deal with the smell by neutralizing it and by killing bacteria.

- Antiperspirants, on the other hand, try to prevent sweating by blocking the pores using aluminum. Without sweat, the bacteria cannot metabolize proteins and fatty acids that cause body odor.

Antiperspirants: The over-the-counter drug

You might be surprised to learn that the antiperspirant you use daily is in fact an over-the-counter (OTC) drug. As mentioned above, **antiperspirants work by clogging, closing, or blocking the pores with aluminum salts in order to prevent the release of sweat**, effectively changing the function of the body. Antiperspirants are considered to be drugs because they affect the physiology of the body.

Because antiperspirants are drugs, they are regulated by the Food and Drug Administration (FDA). Consequently, every antiperspirant sold in the US has a Drug Identification Number, which you can find on the label. A document called "monograph" states requirements for categories of non-prescription drugs such as antiperspirants. It defines, for example, what ingredients may be used and for what purpose. If the standards of the OTC monograph are met, premarket approval of a potentially new OTC product is not necessary.

Antiperspirants contain many active and inactive ingredients. Aluminum is the most common one. Most antiperspirants also contain paraben, an ingredient that is also used in deodorants.

Deodorants

As mentioned above, deodorants deal with body odor by neutralizing the smell and by killing the bacteria that metabolize the proteins and fatty acids that occur naturally in sweat.

In the last decade, one particular ingredient in conventional deodorants has become controversial: paraben, a widely used preservative.

Both antiperspirants and deodorants are considered to be safe by the FDA, the American Cancer Society, the National Cancer Institute and the Mayo Clinic—but within the holistic health field, we know better.

There are some very safe alternatives to dangerous, cancer-causing deodorants—many of which you can create yourself!

THE NATURAL SOLUTION

Your underarms are a very sensitive area: your lymph area, where white blood cells are made. Stop putting that toxic deodorant or antiperspirant under your arms! Apply therapeutic, natural essential oils instead.

Many **antibacterial essential oils** can be applied directly under the armpits for effective protection, natural fragrance and herbal health benefits. Antibacterial essential oils are extremely effective at eliminating underarm odor, but do not stop perspiration.

Listed below are some favorite solutions. Simply apply 3 to 5 drops of undiluted oil to your fingertips and rub it under each armpit as needed. The oils will do their job for 6 to 12 hours. Re-apply throughout the day when needed.

Not only does this method keep you somewhat dry, but the oils add benefits to the bloodstream and act as antibacterial agents. If you need something stronger, then re-apply more often throughout the day. Another option is to use a readymade deodorant product like the Aroma Guard© natural deodorant available from Young Living that will keep you protected. (See index for this formula).

REAL GREENING: YOUR DEODORANTS

Print out this handy guide for your home reference.

Cypress essential oil

- Helps to improve circulation, anti-infectious, strengthens blood capillaries, lymph cleansing.

- Fragrance creates a sense of security and grounding, helps heal emotional trauma, calms, and soothes anger, helps life flow better.

Gentle Baby essential oil blend

- Soothing, good for dry skin, revitalizing, anti-infectious.

- Fragrance is relaxing and balancing, restores confidence, relieves anxiety & stress, helps with depression.

Geranium essential oil

- Good for skin care, anti-infectious, anti-inflammatory, antibacterial, anti-fungal, improves blood flow, liver and pancreas stimulant, dilates bile ducts for liver detoxification.

- Fragrance helps release negative memories and eases nervous tension. Also helps to relieve depression, anxiety and frustration.

Lavender essential oil

- Good for skin conditions, anti-septic, anti-fungal.

- Fragrance is calming, relaxing, balancing; reduces depression, increases cognitive performance.

Palmarosa essential oil

- Antibacterial, anti-fungal, antiviral, stimulates new skin cell growth, good for skin problems.

- Fragrance creates a feeling of security, reduces stress and tension, and promotes recovery from nervous exhaustion.

Patchouli essential oil

- Anti-microbial, reduces fluid retention, relieves itching, good for skin conditions.

- Fragrance is relaxant, clarifies thoughts, helps to discard obsessions, jealousy and insecurities.

Rosewood essential oil

- Antibacterial, antifungal, antiviral.

- Fragrance is empowering and emotionally stabilizing.

Sandalwood essential oil

- Good for skin conditions, anti-viral, anti-microbial.

- Fragrance helps to remove negative programming from the cells; stimulates the pineal gland – releasing melatonin (that is antitumoral and an immune-stimulant); and is grounding and stabilizing.

Vetiver essential oil

- Great for men. Anti-inflammatory, antiseptic, relaxant, good for skin care.

- Fragrance is psychologically grounding, calming, stabilizing; helps stress reduction, recovery from emotional trauma; increases attention.

Ylang Ylang essential oil

- Anti-inflammatory, anti-diabetic, good for skin care, antispasmodic, good for cardiac problems.

- Fragrance helps to balance male/female energies, combats low-self-esteem and anger.

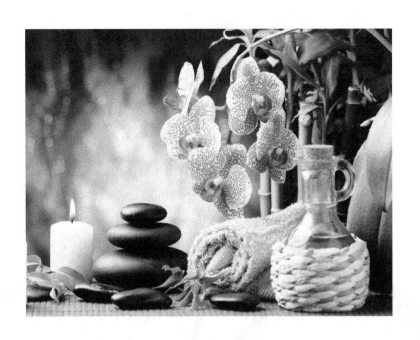

CHAPTER *9*:

Are insects bugging you?

"No need to panic! Take scents-able action with Real Green Essentials©.

CHAPTER 9:

Spring and summertime means spending time outdoors! Stings and bites from insects are common for many of us and can make being outdoors unpleasant. Stings often result in redness and swelling in the injured area. Sometimes a sting can cause a life-threatening allergic reaction. **Considering both multiple stings and allergic reactions to single stings, insects actually harm or even kill (in rare cases) more than three times as many North Americans as snakes do.**

The insect responsible for the largest number of severe allergic reactions is the yellow jacket wasp. When I experienced a yellow jacket wasp sting a few years ago, I knew I was in trouble. As I opened the trunk of my car one summer's day, I was immediately attacked by an unwanted visitor. I raised my hand to protect myself and ended up being stung on my right thumb.

Not only was the sting painful, but my thumb began to swell. I immediately entered my car to search for my lavender oil which luckily I carry with me most of the time. **Dripping a drop or two on my thumb, I observed the most amazing transformation before my eyes. My thumb, swollen to the size of a small marble, shrank to its normal size in**

seconds—pain free! It was a marvel and certainly a life saver that day for me. And I know that it may just do that for you or someone you know.

Insect bites can be a quick way to destroy a fun time or your holiday time, especially with the risk of the West Nile Virus that has sprung up all over the country in recent years. The risk is more serious for the elderly, young children or people with compromised immune systems. With the right natural remedies, you can protect yourself and your family from summer time bugs. A few tips and natural formulas are given below to help you avoid the pesticides.

WHAT ARE THE DANGERS OF COMMON BUG REPELLENTS?

The common recommendation that is made for outdoor use, in particular, is DEET (N,N-diethyl-m-toluamide) – the most widely used repellent. **DEET is a registered pesticide. It is a member of the toluene chemical family. Toluene is a hazardous waste and an endocrine disruptor as well as a potential cancer causing agent.**

A recent study suggests that DEET could interfere with your nervous system. DEET can also cause severe skin irritation, blistering, and burning in some individuals. Most often, DEET is used with other pesticides, creating highly dangerous combinations.

In one animal study, DEET was found to cause behavioral problems when combined with the insect repellent permethrin. Permethrin in itself is quite toxic, and especially to cats. It is a member of the synthetic pyrethroid family, known as neurotoxins (which mean it will be damaging to the pineal and pituitary glands). **The EPA has even classified this chemical carcinogenic: It causes lung tumors, liver tumors, immune system problems and chromosomal abnormalities.**

Permethrin and DEET are also damaging to the environment, especially toxic to bees and aquatic life. The chemicals build up in rivers and streams, damaging the environment. Rodale reports that a U.S. Geological Survey sampling of stream water quality detected DEET in 73 percent of sampled waterways, some of which may feed into drinking-water supplies. **What are we doing to our environment and ourselves?**

Environmental health reports that applied topically, up to 56 percent of DEET penetrates intact human skin and 17 percent is absorbed into the bloodstream. Reports confirmed that blood concentrations of about 3 mg per litre were detected several hours after DEET repellent was applied to skin in the prescribed fashion. DEET is also absorbed by the gut.

A 2013 study suggests that **mosquitoes can at least temporarily overcome or adapt to the repellent effect of DEET after an initial exposure**, representing a non-genetic behavioral change. What are the implications? Is this not a similar issue to the drug-resistant "superbug" bacterium that is also prevailing globally?

Sadly, DEET is still widely used. According to the EPA, every year, approximately **one-third** of the U.S. population is expected to use DEET.

AVOID other harmful chemicals in repellents—like *Dimethyl phthalate (DEP)* which has been linked to testicular cancer and cell mutation.

GREENING OUR BUG REPELLENTS

The more that you and others realize the dangers of DEET and other pesticides, while educating yourselves about the **dozens of green mosquito and bug repellents available**, then the more you and others will all lessen the chemical burden for our planet. DEET can become a toxin of the past.

Natural oils as insect repellents

Two botanical repellents which performed particularly well in a Florida study were a **lemon eucalyptus essential oil (providing 120 minutes of protection) and Citronella oil (30-40 minutes of protection).** The authors note that the oils just need to be applied more often.

The CDC also reports that **lemon eucalyptus oil** also known **as *Eucalyptus citriadora* provides protection similar to repellents with low concentrations of DEET.** The CDC has given its approval for lemon eucalyptus as an effective repellent.

What insects cause itchy or painful bites?

Mosquito bites, harvest mites (also called chiggers), fleas, and bedbugs usually cause itchy, red bumps. The size of the swelling can vary from a dot to a centimetre (half inch). Mosquito bites near the eye usually cause serious swelling for multiple days.

Clues that a bite is a mosquito bite are itchiness, a central raised dot in the swelling, and presence of the bite on a surface not covered by clothing. Some mosquito bites in sensitive children form hard lumps that last for months. In contrast to mosquitoes, fleas and bedbugs don't fly; therefore, they crawl under clothing to nibble. Flea bites often turn into little blisters in young children.

Bites of horseflies, deerflies, gnats, fire ants, harvester ants, blister beetles, and centipedes usually cause a painful, red bump. Within a few hours, fire ant bites change to blisters or pimples.

Neem oil blended with coconut or jojoba oil is another plant-based traditional Indian insect repellent. Catnip and thyme essential oils were found to be more effective in warding off mosquitoes and other bugs than DEET.

Dr. Joseph Mercola reported another study that showed cinnamaldehyde, the chief constituent found in **cinnamon leaf oil**, to be effective as a pesticide— without the risk of negative health and environmental consequences.

Essential oils are the active ingredient in many brand-name products. Of course, using the real natural product that is unhampered by chemical solvents and the like is the best alternative, giving you the most in usage and safety. Just a reminder: There are many essential oil companies. Not all essential oils are created equal. Purity and quality is absolutely critical in order to obtain maximum results and safety. My choice (as explained in Chapter 2) is the use of a therapeutic, genuine; clean all organic essential oil by Young Living Company.

More bug-repelling ideas:

- Eliminate breeding grounds by removing sources of standing water (flowerpots, kiddie pools, garbage bins, birdbaths, etc.)

- Use yellow outdoor light bulbs to help reduce mosquito populations at night.

- Use a fan when there is little wind, since mosquitoes are not strong flyers and the wind disturbs the chemical sweat coming off your bodies.

- Plant mosquito-repelling plants like lemon balm, catnip, basil and lemon geraniums around outdoor sitting areas.

- Encourage mosquito predators like bats, dragonflies, birds, frogs and beetles, which can help reduce mosquito populations.

- Mosquitoes are also attracted by carbon dioxide, lactic acid and other body chemicals, as well as your body heat and sweat, and can sense these chemicals from 25-35 meters. Be aware beer drinking increases carbon dioxide.

- Use essential oils either singularly or any formula mix below prior to your outings, this will help avoid the need for any chemical repellent.

INSECT REPELLENT AND BUG BITE TREATMENTS

Make your own homemade insect repellent sprays and lotions, and treat itchy or painful bug bites without chemicals.

- As a general rule, use **Lemongrass or Citronella** to keep insects at bay: Diffuse into the air, infuse paper strips at the windows, on light bulbs, etc.

- Use **lavender** oil to deter insects from landing on your skin.

- Olive oil is in itself an insect repellent. So mix 5 tablespoons **olive oil** with equal amounts of **cinnamon oil** (a powerful repellent) and mix it well. Will keep mosquitoes away from you.

- Dab oils neat on neck and legs, or use a spray bottle.

- Ankles are a prime target for mosquitoes. Cover the ankles with cotton socks and add a drop of **Lavender or Purification** to the tops of the socks. Put drops of essential oils on bottom of pant legs.

All-purpose insect spray and lotion:

To make a spray, use a base of witch hazel, olive oil, or vodka. Add one or a combination of the oils listed below, at a ratio of 10 parts base to 2 parts essential oil. Mix in a spray bottle.

- Lemongrass
- Eucalyptus citriadora (most effective)

- Thyme

- Peppermint

- Lavender

- Cinnamon

- Cedarwood

- Citronella (most effective)

- Purification Blend (most effective)

To make a repellent lotion, add 120 drops of the above listed oils to two ounces of distilled water in a deep mixing bowl. Using a wire whip, beat the mixture quickly while gradually adding two ounces of olive oil. Store the mixture in a jar or bottle and use as needed. Especially useful while hiking.

Insect Deterrent
- Combine 4 drops Thyme, 8 drops Lemongrass, 4 drops Lavender, 4 drops Peppermint, 8 drops Lemon Eucalyptus and 4 drops Cinnamon oil. Mix together and apply neat, or add to a 8-ounce bottle with distilled water.

House and garden bug spray - Green Pesticides
- 3 drops of Spearmint and 3 drops Orange oil mixed in 2 quarts water. Spray on plants in the house and outside to keep the bugs and aphids away.

- Mix equal parts of vinegar with a cap of Thieves Household Cleaner concentrate in a quart of water. Spray on plants.

- **Preparation for another natural- green pesticide**

- Fill an 8-oz. spray bottle with distilled water

- Add 1 ½ tablespoons of liquid dish soap- preferably Thieves household cleaner

- Add 3–4 drops of each of the oils listed below:

- Spearmint essential oil,

- Citronella essential oil

- Lavender essential oil

- Blue tansy essential oil

- Cedarwood essential oil essential oil

Mix and spray generously on plants, fruits, and vegetables

– Thanks to Marco Colindres III, YL Product Marketing Manager for the above recipe listed on the Young Living website.

- Spearmint essential oil can help deter ants and aphids

- Citronella essential oil can help deter gnats and mosquitoes

- Lavender essential oil can help deter fleas, moths and flies

- Blue tansy essential oil can help deter flies

- Cedarwood essential oil can help deter snails and slugs

Fungus on plants:

Lemon and orange essential oils can help reduce fungi from growing on plants- by simply adding 3-4 drops to a 8 oz bottle of water.

Mosquito repellents

- Combine in equal parts: Citronella, *Eucalyptus citriadora* (Lemon Eucalyptus), Basil, Lemongrass, Thyme, Patchouli and Cinnamon oil.

- Combine Lemon, Peppermint, Eucalyptus, Lemongrass and Citronella.

- Young Living Oil Blends: Lemongrass with Citronella, Idaho Tansy with floral water, Purification, Thieves or Melrose.

Oils for other insects

- Moth Repellent: Patchouli

- Horse-Fly repellent: Idaho tansy (create floral water and spray)

- Aphid repellent: Mix 10 drops spearmint and 15 drops orange essential oils in 2 quarts salt water. Shake well and spray on plants.

- Cockroach repellent: Mix 10 drops peppermint and 5 drops cypress in ½ cup salt water. Shake well and spray where roaches live.

- Silverfish repellent: Eucalyptus radiata, Eucalyptus citriadora

Treatments and Remedies

- Reduce irritation by making your own lavender-peppermint spray: To one cup distilled water, add 20 drops lavender and 20 drops peppermint oils. This will help to reduce bite-induced itching and infection.

- Disinfect bites by combining 10 drops Lavender with 20 drops Thyme and 10 drops Lemon Eucalyptus. Or add 8 drops each of these oils, with 5 drops Oregano, to a bowl of water for washing the skin.

- Take a few drops of Oregano, Longevity or Exodus oils internally several times throughout the day, with water.

Bee sting treatments

- Single oils: Lavender, Idaho Tansy.   Blends: Purification, Melrose, Pan Away

- Mix 2 drops Lavender, 1 drop Helichrysum, 1 drop Chamomile, 1 drop Wintergreen.

- Apply 1 or 2 drops Purification, Melrose, Lavender, or Idaho Tansy on location. Repeat until the venom spread has stopped.

- Apply Lavender with or without one or more of the single oils listed, 2 to 3 times daily until redness abates.

Flick or scrape stinger out with credit card or knife, taking care not to squeeze the venom sack.

Chigger (Mite) Bites

- Use Lavender, Tea tree (melaleuca) or Purification blend. Massage 2 to 6 drops of undiluted oil on location, 3-5 times daily.

Ticks

- Use single oils of Thyme, Oregano, Peppermint, RC Blend or Purification blend. Apply Thyme oil to tick to loosen from skin. Then apply Purification on site to detoxify wound. Apply 1 drop Peppermint every 5 minutes for 50 minutes to reduce pain and infection.

Brown Recluse Spider Bite:

The bite of this spider causes painful redness and blistering which progresses to a gangrenous slough of the affected area. **Seek immediate medical attention** and use this treatment in the interim.

- Spider bite blend: 1 drop Lavandin, 1 drop Helichrysum, 1 drop Melrose—or use Purification Blend. Apply one drop of either of the 2 above blends until reaching medical treatment.

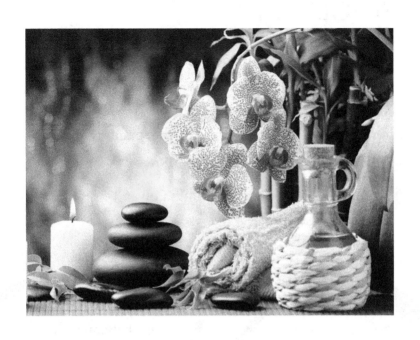

INDEX OF

essential oils and their benefits

*THESE SUGGESTED USES APPLY
ONLY TO THE USE OF*

*THERAPEUTIC GRADE, AUTHENTIC
YOUNG LIVING ESSENTIAL OILS.*

SINGLE OILS

Blue Cypress (found in special blend Brain Power)

Blue Cypress (*Callitris intratropica*) has anti-inflammatory, antiviral, insect repellent, and sedative properties. It is a stimulant to the amygdala, pineal gland, pituitary gland and hypothalamus.

Cedarwood (also found in Brain Power, Inspiration)
**For your pineal gland!

Cedarwood (*Cedrus atlantica*) is high in sesquiterpenes, which can stimulate the limbic part of the brain. Stimulates the pineal gland, which releases melatonin, improves thoughts and cognition. It has a warm, balsamic, woody aroma. It is relaxing and soothing when used for massage, and has long been used as a beneficial ingredient in cosmetic preparations for oily skin.

Household Uses

- Insecticide: Cedar Wood Oil has long been in use as a mosquito and insect repellent. If used in vaporizers, it drives away mosquitoes, flies and other insects from the home.

- Fungicide: Cedar Wood Oil has good fungicidal properties and may be employed to cure fungal infections, both external and internal.

- Dryer: To create great smelling laundry, apply a few drops of your favorite essential oil to a wash cloth and add to the laundry during drying.

- Floors: mix 10 - 15 drops in water and use to wash wooden floors.

Other Uses

- Antibacterial, antiseptic, anti-spasmodic, tonic, astringent, diuretic, insecticide, sedative and fungicide.

- Tonic: Cedar Wood Oil can be used as a health tonic as it tones the organic systems and stimulates metabolism. It tones up muscles, skin, nervous system, stomach, digestive system and brain functions

- Stimulates the limbic region of the brain, especially the pineal gland

- Helps soothe toothache, strengthens grip of gums on teeth and protect them from falling

- Tightens loosened muscles and gives a feeling of firmness

Citronella (found in special blend Purification)

Household Uses

- Insect repellent: Add to strips of blotting paper and hang in closets, or mix in water and create your own spray

- Deodorant

- Insecticidal: Mix a solution 8-10 drops in gallon of water and spray around garden plants

Other Uses

- Antibacterial, antifungal, anti-inflammatory, antiseptic, antispasmodic

- Treat intestinal parasites, digestive and menstrual problems and stimulant

- Alleviate headaches, respiratory infections, neuralgia, fatigue, oily skin

Clary Sage

Clary Sage (*Salvia sclarea*) has anti-convulsive, anti-fungal, sedative, soothing and nerve tonic properties. It is balancing to the hormones, and enhances the circulation.

Cypress

Household Uses

- Insect repellent: Mix 10-15 drops in a small spray bottle filled with water

- Air freshener: Add to a diffuser or potpourri

- Deodorize shoes: Impregnate strips of blotting paper and place in shoes overnight

- Furniture polish: Add to vegetable oil to make your own furniture polish

Other Uses

- Anti-infectious, antibacterial, antimicrobial, and strengthens blood capillaries

- Improves circulation and supports the nerves and intestines. Mostly used for circulatory system

- Arthritis, bronchitis, cramps, haemorrhoids, insomnia, intestinal parasites, menopausal problems, menstrual pain, pancreas insufficiencies, pulmonary infections, rheumatism, spasms, tuberculosis, throat problems, varicose veins, fluid retention, strengthen blood capillary walls, reduce cellulite, bleeding gums, coughs

Eucalyptus Globulus

Household Uses

- Laundry: Add 20 to 25 drops with the wash water to eliminate dust mites

- Use for wiping counters, toilets, sinks etc.

- Kitchen disinfectant for fridge, garbage area etc.

- Powerful insect repellent

Other uses

- Antiviral, antibacterial, antifungal, antiaging

- Decongestant, respiratory/sinuses, arthritis, sore muscles, many other uses

- Colds and coughs: Diffuse it in a diffuser, or add to hot water and let sit

- Contains a high amount of eucalyptol, a powerful antimicrobial agent used in mouthwash

- Trees planted to help to stop the spread of malaria in Africa

- 2 percent eucalyptus oil sprayed in the air will kill 70 percent of airborne staph bacteria

Helichrysum (found in special blend Brain Power)
**For your pineal gland!

Helichrysum (*Helichrysum italicum*) is a powerful natural anti-inflammatory. It also improves circulation and may help cleanse the blood. Helps to **chelate heavy metals and specifically will chelate and <u>detoxify fluoride</u> and <u>petrochemicals </u>**from your **pineal gland.**

Household Uses:

- Add 2-3 drops to a spray bottle with water and spritz bed sheets.

- Use in your bath water: Mix 2-3 drops with sea salt or Epsom salts.

Other Uses:

- Anti-inflammatory, antibacterial, anti-fungal, antispasmodic, detoxifier, chelates chemicals and toxins, regenerates nerves

- The fragrance is uplifting to the subconscious

- Oil of Helichrysum is fantastic for circulatory conditions, blood clots, liver and bruises. Its regenerative power makes it fantastic for skin and any skin conditions.

- Create a salt rub: Add 3 drops to ½ cup of sea salt with 2 tbsp of almond oil. Rub a small handful over skin while showering

- Natural sunscreen: Mix 10 drops with 100 drops of sesame oil or olive oil as your natural sun block

Idaho Balsam Fir

**HIGHLY RECOMMENDED for your pineal gland!

Idaho Balsam Fir helps to regenerate DNA telomeres, reduce stress and cortisol-stress hormone production and is helpful for fatigue.

Household Uses:

- Add drops to a spray bottle and spritz linen, wardrobe, drawers

- Use as a potpourri or deodorizer

- Add drops to a cotton ball and place in drawers

Other Uses:

- Anti-inflammatory, antiseptic, astringent, expectorant, sedative, tonic and anticoagulant

- Spiritual Influence: Calming to the body and stimulating to the mind; Grounding

- Balsam Fir oil is also very soothing to rheumatic pain and great for muscles (or joints and tendons) that have been overworked or are tired.

- Used traditionally for fever and any kind of respiratory or sinus infections. Helpful to diffuse

Idaho Blue Spruce

**HIGHLY RECOMMENDED for your pineal gland!

Idaho Blue Spruce Essential Oil is grounding and provides a feeling of deep peace and security. It helps us to open our heart by providing a sense of security and trust in who we are. Brings peace to the mind and relaxes the body. Its aromatic influences also help open and release emotional blocks, bringing a feeling of balance and peaceful security.

Household Uses:

- Add drops to a spray bottle and spritz linen, wardrobe, drawers

- Use as a potpourri or deodorizer

- Use in your diffuser or add drops to create your own spritzer bottle

- Add drops to a cotton ball and place in drawers

Other Uses:

- The refreshing, invigorating, and strengthening properties of blue spruce also have a long history of use in the sauna, steam bath, and as an additive to baths or massage oils.

- May help relieve muscle tension. Relaxes, soothes, and calms both body and mind

- Useful to help cleanse cuts, bruises, and skin irritations

- Arthritis and rheumatism, infections (respiratory and sinus), bacterial infection, bronchitis, cough, decongestant, immune depression, muscle tension, sinus infection and congestion, skin conditions, viral infection and cut and wound healing

Idaho Tansy

Idaho Tansy (*Tanacetum vulgare*) has antiviral, antibacterial, anti-infectious and anti-inflammatory properties. It is supportive to the immune system. Helps skin problems; strengthens kidneys, heart, joints and digestive system

Jasmine Absolute (found in special blend Into The Future)

Jasmine Absolute (*Jasminum officinale*) has antidepressant and antispasmodic properties. It is emotionally uplifting, unblocks past blocks, alleviates nervous exhaustion.

Juniper

Juniper (*Juniperus osteosperma*) elevates spiritual awareness, creates feelings of love and peace. Has antiseptic, cleanser, detoxifier, diuretic and antispasmodic properties. It is a detoxifier and a cleanser.

Lavender

Lavandula angustifolia is the most versatile of all essential oils. It has analgesic and anti-spasmodic properties. It helps relieve stress, sore muscles, menstrual cramps and nervous tension in the body.

Household Uses

- Antiseptic and antifungal, disinfectant
- All-around household addition to your cleansing
- Add to your laundry
- Air freshener: Add to your cedar chips; Impregnate blotting paper to hang in closets, cupboards, etc.
- Insect repellent and treatment for insect bites
- Great to use in a spray bottle for counter tops, wiping cupboards, refrigerators etc.
- First aid in the kitchen: excellent for burns

Other Uses

- Antiseptic, analgesic, antitumor, anticonvulsant, sedative, anti-inflammatory, cleans wounds (prevents build-up of excess sebum, a skin oil that bacteria feed on)
- Promotes tissue regeneration; Therapeutic-grade lavender has been highly regarded for the skin.
- Relaxing effects, for high blood pressure, sunburns, insomnia

- May be used to cleanse cuts, bruises and skin irritations.

- Fragrance is calming, relaxing and balancing– physically and emotionally.

- Hives, dandruff, hair loss, allergies, convulsions, herpes, headaches, indigestion, insomnia, high blood pressure, menopausal conditions, nausea, phlebitis, tumours, premenstrual conditions

- Minimizes scarring, acne, dermatitis, eczema, psoriasis, rashes, stretch marks

- MAY HELP: arthritis, asthma, bronchitis, depression, earaches, heart palpitations, high blood pressure, insect bites, laryngitis, nervous tension, respiratory infections, rheumatism and throat infections

Lemon

**HIGHLY RECOMMENDED for your pineal gland!

Lemon oil, via its vapors alone, will help to cleanse your pineal by digesting the hydrocarbon deposits that block or cloud this gland.

Read more about Lemon oil's amazing capabilities in Chapter 5.

Household Uses:

- Add one teaspoon of lemon essential oil to one cup mineral oil for an effective furniture polish.

- For general household cleaning purposes, it works well for removing gum, wood stain, oil, and grease spots.

- Add a few drops to your dishwasher for spot free dishes.

- Diffuse to freshen your home.

- Add a few drops to a spray bottle to deodorize and sterilize the air and counter tops.

- Add ten drops to a cotton ball and place it inside your vacuum cleaner

- Use 6 drops of Lemon oil and 6 drops of Purification oil in a squirt bottle mixed with distilled water to help in the bathroom as an air freshener.

- Add drops of lemon with baking soda to wash your kitchen sink and counter tops.

- Add to baking soda for scrubs and washing counter tops, tubs and many other tips already presented earlier in this book.

- Diffuse to freshen your home or add a few drops to a spray bottle to deodorize and sterilize the air.

- Add ten drops to a cotton ball and place inside your vacuum cleaner

Lemongrass

**For your pineal gland!

Lemongrass helps to promote psychic awareness.

Household Uses

- Fabulous antiseptic, fights salmonella and food poisoning

- Purification: Helps to purify the air of nasty smells and bacteria. Use in your diffuser or air freshener.

- Used for digestion

- Has powerful antifungal properties

- Antibacterial, antiparasitic

Other Uses

- Supports digestion, tones and helps regenerate connective tissues and ligaments, dilates blood vessels, strengthens vascular walls, promotes lymph flow

- Anti-inflammatory and sedative

- Bladder infections, digestion disturbances, parasites, torn ligaments, edema, fluid retention, kidney disorders and varicose veins

- MAY HELP: improve circulation, digestion, eyesight, Combat headaches, infections, respiratory problems, sore throats and fluid retention

} Special note: In June 2008, an essential oil-sponsored study[9] was published in the ***Flavor and Fragrance Journal.*** Researchers tested 91 single essential oils with 78 of them that showed zones of inhibition against MRSA. Sixty-four blends were tested and 52 showed inhibition. With the majority of MRSA studies being done on ***Melaleuca alternifolia,*** it was somewhat surprising to find that **the most *effective single oil against MRSA in this study was lemongrass,* which completely inhibited all MRSA growth on the plate.**

} **The only other oil or blend to completely inhibit MRSA was the Young Living blend called R.C.**

Lime

Household Uses

- Great as an air freshener: Invigorates the mind and body

- Diffuse; use in your dishwasher or your wash: The aroma banishes the feeling of apathy, anxiety and depression

- Apply a few drops to your dust cloth

- Insect deterrent: Apply on blotting strips and hang indoors or out

- Fruit or veggie wash: Add 3 to 5 drops of citrus or Lime oil to up to 1 gallon of water in a bowl, mix well, then use as a wash for your fruits and vegetables. Dry well. Will also help prevent premature molding or rotting (protects them from getting spoiled from infection by microbes).

- Carpet deodorizer: Apply 20 drops to 1 cup baking soda. Use a hole punch to punch several holes in the lid of a glass jar. Sprinkle on carpet. Wait ½ to 1 hour then vacuum. Can use other oils for various aromas.

Other Uses

- Applied externally, it protects skin and wounds from infections and helps them heal quickly. It can be used in dilution for applying on scalp to protect hair from various infections, lice etc.

- Can be helpful for arthritis, rheumatism and poor circulation: Relieves pain in muscles and joints, while revitalizing a tired mind

- Supports a healthy digestive system

- May aid in weight management and with cellulite

- Good bactericide. Can be used in treatment of food poisoning, diarrhoea, typhoid and cholera which are caused by bacteria.

- Provides astringent and toning benefits and antioxidants on the skin, which may reduce dark spots due to aging, oily skin and acne

- Useful to cool fevers associated with colds, sore throats and flu and aids the immune system while easing coughs bronchitis and sinusitis, as well as helping asthma

- Beneficial to the immune system

- Eases infection in the respiratory tract

- Consumed, it helps to relieve microbial infection in colon, urinary tract, kidneys, genitals etc.

- Further, it can aid internal bacterial infections like in colon, stomach, intestines and urinary tract as well as external infections on skin, ears, eyes and in wounds.

Melissa (found in the Brain Power blend)

Melissa or Lemon Balm (*Melissa officinalis*) has antiviral, anti-inflammatory, antidepressant and relaxant properties. It is calming and uplifting and used for depression.

Myrtle (found in special blend Inspiration)

Myrtle (*Myrtus communis*) has a clear, fresh, herbaceous scent, similar to eucalyptus. Supportive of the respiratory system, skin, and hair, it has been researched for its effects on glandular imbalances and its soothing effects when inhaled. Is energizing, inspiring, elevating. It is also helpful for meditation and lifting the spirit.

Mugwort (found in special blend Inspiration)

Mugwort was used traditionally under pillows to produce vivid dreams.

Orange Oil

**For your pineal gland!

Orange Essential Oil (*Citrus sinensis*) is elevating to the mind and body and brings joy and peace. A 1995 Mie University study documented the ability of citrus fragrances to combat depression and boost immunity.

Household Uses

- Disinfectant for toilets, laundry room, kitchen, etc.

- Mix in a spray bottle to disinfect fruit/vegetables

- Use for countertops/cutting boards: Sterilizes surfaces, kills microbes, disinfectant

- Add to your dishwasher

- Air freshener: Orange brings peace and happiness to the mind

Other Uses

- Orange may also be used to enhance the flavor of food and water.

- Orange (Citrus sinensis) essential oil has a rich, fruity scent that lifts the spirit while providing a calming influence on the body.

- Anti-tumoral, helps with fluid retention

- Rich in the powerful antioxidant d-limonene: 96 percent limonene and aids in maintaining normal cellular regeneration.

- Great for fat cells- cellulite and tightening the skin

Oregano

(*Origanum vulgare, Origanum onites, Origanum minutiflorum, Origanum majorana*): One of the most powerful and versatile essential oils.

Household Uses

- Disinfectant for toilets, laundry room, kitchen, etc.

- Mix in a spray bottle to disinfect fruit/vegetables

- Countertops/cutting boards: Helps to prevent food poisoning, especially when cooking with meat or fish

- Add 1 drop to your dishwashing load

Other Uses:

- Contains strong immune-enhancing and antioxidant properties and supports the respiratory system.

- Oregano may also be used to enhance the flavor of food. Oregano is also a key oil used in the Raindrop Technique, a massage application of essential oils, which is designed to bring about electrical alignment in the body.

- Antibacterial, antifungal, anti- parasitic, anti-microbial, powerful antiviral, antiaging

- Good for infections, arthritis, digestive problems

- Powerful anti-infectious agent for respiratory, intestines, genital, nerves, blood and lymphatics

- Large-spectrum action against bacteria, mycobacteria, fungus, virus and parasites

- Asthma, bronchitis, mental disease, pulmonary tuberculosis, rheumatism (chronic), whooping cough

Palmarosa

**For your pineal gland!

Palmarosa has recently been found to be a neuro-protective-that is it protects your brain.

Household Uses

- Antibacterial, anti-fungal, antiviral, antimicrobial

- Scouring powder: Mix baking soda with 20 drops of Palmarosa

- Laundry: Add 10 -15 drops on damp cloth

- Wash kitchen countertops with cloth soaked with Palmarosa

- Spritz cutting boards with water mixed with Palmarosa

- Deodorize your refrigerator

Other Uses

Palmarosa oil has a variety of therapeutic uses.

- Especially beneficial : Hydrates by helping to retain the moisture in the tissues and maintains the moisture balance

- Stimulates cell regeneration: regulates sebum production, giving it age-defying properties. Aromatherapists love Palmarosa for its skin conditioning properties

- Stimulates new cell growth, regulates oil production, moisturizes and speeds healing.

- Uterine tonic and cardiotonic

- Supportive to the nerves and circulation

- Additionally, Palmarosa oil is great for the digestive system, and was added to Indian curry dishes and West African meat dishes to destroy bacteria and aid digestion.

- For fatigue, nervousness, physical exhaustion, depression, stress and stress-related conditions

- Wow—how about a clean bathroom smelling of roses and reducing stress all at the same time!

- MAY HELP: candida, cardiovascular system, circulation, digestion, infection, nervous system and rashes

Rosewood (found in special blend Inspiration)

Rosewood (*Aniba roseodora*) has a relaxing, empowering effect. It is very grounding and strengthening. This oil is soothing, creates elasticity, and helps the skin rid itself of irritations and problems, such as Candida. It is anti-infectious, antibacterial, antifungal, antiviral, and antiparasitic.

Sacred Frankincense

**HIGHLY RECOMMENDED for your pineal gland!

Frankincense (*Boswellia sacra*) is considered holy anointing oil in the Middle East and has been used in religious ceremonies for thousands of years. High in sesquiterpenes, it helps stimulate the limbic part of the brain, which elevates the mind, helping to overcome stress and despair. It is used in European medicine to combat depression.

Household Uses:

- Add drops to a spray bottle and spritz linen, wardrobe, drawers

- Impregnate blotting paper with drops of Sacred Frankincense and hang in closets

- Use for your meditation or relaxation practices

- Use in your diffuser or add drops to create your own spritzer bottle

- Use as a potpourri or deodorizer

- Add drops to a cotton ball and place in drawers

- Add a few drops to your laundry or your dryer

- Add to your dishwashing along with the Thieves household cleaner

Other uses:

- Anti-cancerous, anti-catarrhal, anti-depressant, anti-infectious, anti-tumoral, antiseptic, expectorant, immune-stimulant, muscle relaxant and sedative

- Asthma, cancer, depression, infection (colds, coughs, pneumonia, respiratory, staph, strep), immune stimulant, inflammation, muscles, nervous conditions, supports the nervous system, stress, ulcers and vertigo.

- Spiritual Influence: Will help to release feelings of unworthiness and insecurity and disconnection from our soul.

Sandalwood

**For your pineal gland!

Sandalwood (*Santalum album*) is extremely high in sesquiterpenes which helps to stimulate the pineal gland and limbic brain. Used traditionally in yoga and meditation and may help to remove negative programming from the cells. Has anti-depressant, astringent, aphrodisiac and sedative properties. It is calming and emotionally balancing and is used for depression and stress.

Household Uses:

- Use as a deodorizer

- Diffuse in the room for relaxation and/or meditation

- Add several drops to a spray bottle with water and spritz bed sheets and towels. Enjoy the fresh and invigorating aroma

Other Uses:

- Antidepressant, antiviral, antitumoral, immune stimulant, calming, astringent, antiseptic

- Helps to improve balance and harmony

- Creates deep relaxation of the nervous system and used for centuries to enhance meditation.

- Aphrodisiac, sedative, tonic, bronchial dilator

Spruce

*** **For your pineal gland**

Spruce (*Picea mariana*) helps to open and release emotional blocks, bringing about a feeling of balance and grounding. Traditionally, spruce oil was believed to possess the frequency of prosperity. Spruce is anti-infectious, antiseptic, and anti-inflammatory.

Household Uses

- Air freshener: Opens the third eye. The Lakota Indians used spruce to strengthen their ability to communicate with the Great Spirit.

- Add to cedar chips to make your own potpourri

- Add to strips of blotting paper and hang in closets

- Great addition to make your furniture polish

- Put spruce oil on a cotton ball or tissues and place them in your car, home or work environment. Especially helpful over air vents and in hotel rooms

- Sprinkle a few drops on a damp cloth and place near an intake duct for your heating and cooling system to vent the aroma throughout your home

Other Uses

- Asthma, bronchitis, mental disease, pulmonary tuberculosis, rheumatism (chronic), whooping cough

- General tonic and immune stimulant

- Antispasmodic, anti-infectious, anti-parasitic, antiseptic, anti-inflammatory

- Respiratory infections, digestion problems, balance metabolism, viral and bacterial pneumonia, and strengthen the vital centers

Tea Tree

Melaleuca alternifolia is highly regarded for its wide range of uses.

Household Uses

- Protects from radiation: Can be used in a spray around your office desk (computers)

- Add a few drops to a potpourri and place near computer, TV and other EMF exposures. Especially beneficial: Add 20 drops to a bowl of peat moss and hazel nuts. Replace every 3-6 months

- Cleansing: Add to your wash cloths, laundry rooms, kitchen

- Anti-infectious, powerful antibacterial, antifungal, anti-viral, antiseptic due to its high terpinenol-4 content

Other Uses

- Immunostimulant: Supports the immune system

- Beneficial for the skin: Acne, sores, fungal infections

- Antiparasitic, anti-inflammatory, cardio tonic, decongestant of the veins,

- Athletes foot, fungal infections, bronchitis, respiratory infections, gum disease, rash, sore throat, sunburn, tonsillitis and vaginal thrush

- MAY HELP: burns, candida, cold sores, inflammations, viral infections, ingrown nails, warts and wounds

Thyme

Household Uses

- Highly anti-microbial, anti-fungal, anti-viral, anti-parasitic

- Insecticidal

- Kills bacteria; Great to use as a wipe for your refrigerator, counter tops, sinks and cutting boards. Simply add 4 to 5 drops to a small bowl of water, dip your dish cloth and wipe

Other Uses

- Thymol used in mouthwash, vapor rubs

- Anti-spasmodic, anti-rheumatic, antiseptic, bactericidal

- Clears spasm, gives relief from rheumatism by removing toxins

- Protects wounds from infection; heals scars & afterbirth marks

- Expectorant: Helps aid clearing of chest infections and coughs,

- Good for heart's health

- Gives relief from intestinal gas

- Increases urination, makes menstruations regular

Vetiver

**For your pineal gland!

Vetiver essential oil is very grounding and the aroma is very earthy. Vetiver will help to ground you, and will supply oxygen to the pineal gland.

Household Uses:

- Helps relieve stress and emotional trauma. Use as a deodorizer by adding 10 drops to a spray bottle or diffuser.

- Furniture polish: Mix a few drops in an oil/vinegar mixture to make your own polish

- For a fireplace or campfire: Create an enhanced earthy aroma by placing several drops of Vetiver on a log before placing it in the fire.

Other Uses:

- Antiseptic, circulatory tonic, relaxant

- Rejuvenating on mature skin: Plumps up sagging skin

- Other uses: absentmindedness, acne, arthritis, ADD, ADHD, attention deficit, autism, coma, depression, hyperactivity, joint stiffness, menstrual cramps, mental fatigue, muscles, muscular dystrophy, pancreatitis, postpartum depression, schizophrenia, sore feet

White Fir (found in special blend Into The Future)

White Fir (*Abies concolor*) has analgesic, antiseptic, sedative and tonic properties. Creates feeling of grounding and anchoring. Empowering. It relaxes the body, while stimulating the mind.

White Lotus (found in special blend Into The Future)

White Lotus (*Nymphaea lotus*) is calming and relaxing. Helps you move forward, overcoming self-defeating thoughts. Brings deep peace and comfort.

Ylang Ylang (found in special blend Into The Future)

Ylang Ylang (*Cananga odorata*) increases relaxation, restores confidence and equilibrium, has antidepressant, antispasmodic and sedative properties. It balances the male and female energies of the body.

SPECIAL BLENDS

Brain Power

**HIGHLY RECOMMENDED for your pineal gland!

Brain Power assists with mental clarity and eliminates "brain fog". One of the causes of brain fog is thought to be the toxicity due to petrochemicals and various other synthetic chemicals. Brain Power dissolves petrochemicals around the glands in the brain and along the spine when used in massage. It increases oxygen around the pineal, pituitary and hypothalamus of the brain.

Improves mental focus and concentration, anti-aging, increases growth hormone and melatonin, sleep apnea, improves memory, forgetfulness, jet lag, nervous and mental fatigue, depression, convulsions, dizziness, epilepsy, fainting, headaches, autism.

Contains: Frankincense, **Helichrysum,** Sandalwood, Cedarwood, Melissa or Lemon Balm, Lavender, **Blue Cypress**

Household Uses:

- Air freshener; Add drops to a spray bottle and spritz linen, wardrobe, drawers

- Add a few drops to a cotton ball and place in your drawers

- Add to a damp cloth for your laundry

- Add to sea salt or Epsom salts for bathing:

- Detox fluoride from the pineal gland: Spritz your face with a mixture of 2 to 3 drops with water in a spray bottle

Citrus Fresh

Citrus Fresh is a special Young Living blend that is composed of lemon, orange, tangerine and grapefruit essential oils. It is a great air purifier and known to clean the air and add freshness to the environment. Japanese research found that diffusing a citrus fragrance in offices improved mental accuracy and concentration by 54 percent!

These oils are high in limonene, a potent anti-oxidant, known to prevent DNA damage. A powerful antiseptic, anti-infectious, anti-parasitic and antispasmodic, Citrus Fresh can also be calming, combat anxiety, nervousness, stress and irritability. It is a great oil friend to have nearby—for cleaning, and for the myriad of physical and mental health benefits that it offers! Use as you would Lemon oil.

Inspiration

**HIGHLY RECOMMENDED for your pineal gland!

The essential oils in this blend are rich in sesquiterpenes. Sesquiterpenes is an aromatic chemical that research has shown to oxygenate the pineal gland, has the ability to cross the blood-brain barrier, to oxygenate the brain, clear out plaques and toxins and help with depression. Can also reverse bladder and kidney infections.

Contains: Cedarwood, Spruce, Rosewood, Sandalwood, Frankincense, Myrtle, Mugwort.

Household Uses:

- Add drops to a spray bottle and spritz linen, wardrobe, drawers

- Impregnate blotting paper with a few drops and hang in closets

- Use for your meditation or relaxation practices

- Use in your diffuser or add drops to create your own spritzer bottle

- Use as a potpourri or deodorizer

- Add drops to a cotton ball and place in drawers

- Add a few drops to your laundry or your dryer

- Add to your dishwashing along with the Thieves household cleaner

Into The Future

**For your pineal gland!

Into the Future was formulated to foster feelings of determination and a pioneering spirit, helping you to leave the past behind so that you can move forward. Rather than accepting mediocrity because of fear of the unknown, using this blend will enhance enjoyment of challenges leading to success.

Contains: Frankincense, Ylang Ylang, Clary Sage, Cedarwood, Jasmine Absolute, Orange, Idaho Tansy, Juniper, White Fir, White Lotus

Carrier Oil: Sweet Almond Oil

Household Uses:

- Add drops to a spray bottle and spritz linen, wardrobe, drawers

- Impregnate blotting paper with a few drops and hang in closets

- Use for your meditation or relaxation practices

- Use in your diffuser or add drops to create your own spritzer bottle

- Use as a potpourri or deodorizer

- Add drops to a cotton ball and place in drawers

- Add a few drops to your laundry or your dryer

- Add to your dishwashing along with the Thieves household cleaner

Melrose

Melrose blend is antiseptic, antibacterial, antifungal, antiparasitic, anti-inflammatory. This blend has antimicrobial effects against superbugs or antibacterial-resistant germs.

Special Use: This blend contains two species of Melaleuca that were found through Dr. Daniel Penoel and Pierre Franchomme Ph.D., research to prevent cellular damage from environmental pollution and potential exposure to radiation.

Contains: Melaleuca alternifolia or Tea Tree Oil, Naouli (Melaleuca Quinquenervia) Rosemary, Clove (*Syzygium aromaticum*, one of the most antimicrobial of all essential oils).

Possible skin sensitivity. If pregnant or under a doctor's care, consult your physician. Dilution recommended for both topical and internal use. Dilute before using on sensitive areas such as the face, neck, genital area, etc. Keep out of reach of children. Avoid using on infants and very small children.

Household Uses

- For topical or aromatic use and cleaning and disinfecting uses. Diffuse or apply topically.

- When diffused, Melrose can help dispel odors, purifies the air

- Even protects against daily radiation bombardment- use around computers, while travelling on airplanes-add 2 drops in the bottom of your shoes

- Use in laundry by adding a few drops to the load

- Wipe counters, sinks by adding to your washing water

- Use in spray bottle mixed with water to spray in refrigerators

Other Uses

- Provides a protective barrier against skin challenges.

- Cleanses and disinfects cuts, scrapes, burns, rashes, bruised tissue & infections

- Regenerates damaged tissue and reduces inflammation

Purification

Purification essential oil blend is a versatile combination of Young Living Therapeutic Grade™ essential oils, created to meet a variety of everyday needs.

Citronella is combined with rosemary, lavendin and lemongrass organic essential oils to cleanse and soothe insect bites, to combat the effects of painful bites from spiders, bees, hornets, and wasps, cuts and scrapes. When diffused, it helps to purify and cleanse the air from environmental impurities, including cigarette smoke and other disagreeable odors. It is very useful to use in the kitchen. Purification can even remove undesirable smells from litter boxes and other sources of odor.

Purification blend is for topical or aromatic use for children over 2, adults and pets. Possible skin sensitivity. If pregnant or under a doctor's care, consult your physician. Dilution not required; suitable for all but the most sensitive skin. Generally safe for children over 2 years of age.[60]

Contains: Citronella, Lemongrass, Rosemary, Melaleuca, Lavandin, Myrtle

With Purification blend, you should replace:

- All aerosol sprays and room deodorizers, linked to asthma and other respiratory issues

- Hand sanitizers, which can cause contact dermatitis, thyroid imbalances, hormonal disruption and antibacterial-resistant germs

- Chemical cleaners (as discussed in Chapter 1) that have been linked to cancer, auto-immune disorders, endocrine imbalances

- Antibacterial creams, used for injuries, cuts, scrapes, or wounds

- Chemical insect repellents, pesticides and more!

Household Uses

- Formulated for diffusing to purify and cleanse the air

- Neutralizes mildew, cigarette smoke and disagreeable odors

- Try adding a few drops to a spray bottle to freshen furniture and carpet.

- Apply topically on location as needed, or diffuse and rub on feet for cleansing.

- Use on bathroom surfaces to clean mildew and hard-water stains.

- Insect repellent: Put 10 drops in 8 oz. spray bottle with water. Spray the body and clothing.

- Pets: repels fleas, aids in cleaning cuts, scrapes,

insect bites and even snake bites, removing foul smells and cleansing.

- For smelly shoes: Put 2 drops of Purification oil on two cotton balls. Place in smelly sneakers to combat odors

- Place a drop of Purification oil on a cotton swab and place on top of your cold water humidifier to clean the air.

Other Uses

- Put a drop of Purification oil on insect bites to cleanse and stop the itching. Excellent in drawing out the toxins even from snake bites

- Apply a drop of Purification oil on blemishes to clear the skin.

- Apply a drop of Purification oil topically over throat area at the onset of a sore throat

- Apply a drop of Purification oil to soothe, cleanse and disinfect a blister, cut or scrape

* **Holy Basil** (*Ocimum sanctum*) **and Basil** (ocimum basilicum)

** **Use for the pineal**

Holy Basil is a cross between Basil oil and Clove oil

Basil oil will give a milder effect than the Tulsi oil but will certainly be very helpful.

Holy Basil or Tulsi as it is called in India is planted in the courtyard of Hindu families as they believe that planting Tulsi will bring peace to the home and its residents. Tulsi is believed to be purifying to the environment. It is also considered to be a 'multi-tasker' oil covering many conditions. There are a number of benefits for this oil. People use Tulsi for seasoning uncooked food to avoid chances of food poisoning.

- Anti-oxidants in Tulsi prevents premature aging thus it enhances longevity

- Tulsi essential oil is used to increase mental health

- Skin diseases like acne and psoriasis are very efficiently treated by Tulsi

- Tulsi has a chemical element called flavanoids that prevents cells from radiation and damage

- Essential oils of Tulsi can also be used to treat conditions of anxiety, depression and stress

Tulsi helps to relax muscles and blood vessels and hence improves the flow of blood in the body as it contains Magnesium.

Likewise, **Basil** (ocimum basilicum) has similar qualities.

It is a stimulant for the mind and the memory. It is useful for soothing stress, mild nervousness, anxiety, depression or instances of mental fatigue. It is a welcomed oil to use when afflicted with the common cold, has anti-microbial and anti-viral properties.

When diluted into a warm bath it will help one to relax by soothing muscle aches and menstrual cramps

- Anti-microbial: kills or inhibits the growth of microorganisms such as bacteria, fungi or protozoan's.

- Anti-spasmodic: prevents or relieves muscle spasms

- Anti-oxidant: combats free radicals to discourage cellular damage or death

- Anti-viral: useful for treating viral infections

- Prevents the formation of gas in the gastrointestinal tract

- Helps with poor memory

- Increases perspiration to regulate body temperature

- Digestive: aids in proper digestion and digestive support

- Stimulates blood flow to the pelvic region and the uterus while stimulating menstruation

- Clears mucus from the lungs, bronchi, and trachea by increasing the amount of secretions which lubricate the respiratory tract.

HOME USES:

Use as in other oils for cleaning, dusting, and as an air freshener

Aroma Guard Deodorant

Aroma Guard Deodorants are **the first natural deodorants formulated exclusively from therapeutic-grade essential oils and all-natural ingredients.** They provide a pleasant and safe alternative to commercial deodorants and are free of propylene glycol, parabens, triclosan and toxic aluminum salts.

Ingredients:

Cocos Nucifera (Coconut) oil, White Beeswax, Pure Vegetable Esters, Zinc Oxide, Tocopherols (Vitamin E), Citrus Medica Limonum (Lemon) Fruit Oil, Pelargonium Graveolens (Geranium)† Flower Oil, Rosmarinus Officinalis (Rosemary)† Leaf Oil, Aniba rosaeodora (Rosewood)† Wood Oil, Lavandula angustifolia (Lavender)† Oil, Melaleuca Alternifolia† (Tea Tree) Leaf Oil, Melaleuca Quinquenervia Oil (Niaouli) Oil and Syzgium Aromaticum (Clove)† Oil.

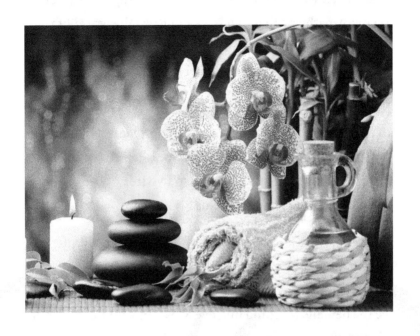

CONCLUSION:

Live real green and thrive!

*Be empowered, educated and
awakened to your true strength!*

Real Green Essentials: Vibrational Cleaning is my offering to you: A pathway that will help you leave the world of toxic chemicals and regain your pure, natural, eco-green and energetically attuned self.

These are the practices and the products that I use every day and they have helped me shed health problems, unhappiness and other symptoms of an unbalanced life. I want to share them with you, so that you can also live free of the chemical shackles that bind so many of us.

Holistic health is the practice of looking at your life as a whole and taking into account all the little things that affect you on a day to day basis. As you adopt this practice, you will see the benefits reaching into every part of your life. Essential oils and all-natural products are your keys to finding balance:

- Removing toxic chemicals from your life, your bloodstream, your body and your brain;

- Stimulating and activating your pineal gland for youthfulness of body, calmness of mind and openness of the spirit;

- Attuning the cells of your body with the high-frequency, vibrational energies distilled from organic, natural herbs and plants;

- Gaining deep psychological and physiological benefits through the aroma's direct connection with your subconscious and conscious brain.

Real Green Essentials- Vibrational Cleaning is a philosophy and a practice that will change your life. By using these products throughout your days, you don't just create a happier, healthier and cleaner home; you actually shift the energy, making your space sacred and spiritually attuned. The effects are joy, calmness and spiritual growth!

In order to help you experience these amazing changes, Real Green Essentials Eco-Consultants will offer you their time and their knowledge. Please contact us to find a consultant near you—or become a consultant for your own area!

We now stand at a very important time for our planet, our wildlife and our human nature. Science is once again discovering the dangers of many of the toxic chemicals we use in our daily lives and the deep benefits of natural solutions. Get involved and "ride the wave of change" into a brighter, healthier future!

At the same time as you step forward into the beauty of a natural, eco-green life, you must also shed the negative and unhealthy influences of the modern world. It's important to develop your awareness of the dangers of electromagnetic radiation, the pervasiveness of cancer-causing chemicals in everyday cleaning and care products, and even the unhealthy additives in foods and air fresheners.

I have spent decades researching and refining the solutions to these problems, even as more toxic chemicals spew forth—

as fast as we can solve problems, new ones arise! And yet, more and more research is proving the simple truth: Nature's power is strong enough to heal us and raise us out of the toxic soup.

I am truly excited to share with you my findings, my favorite products and my own safe, effective methods for cleaning your home, caring for your body and attuning your vibrational energy. Thank you for choosing **Real Green Essentials: Vibrational Cleaning for a Healthy Home**—and a healthy you!

Sabina Devita

Ed.D, DNM, NNCP, DCSJ

About the Author

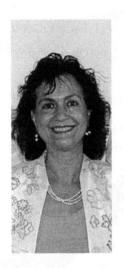

Sabina M. De Vita (Ed.D, D.N.M. N.N.C.P., IASP, CBP, DCSJ) has been a long time environmentalist. When she became ill in the 1980's, with environmental sensitivities, also known as ecological illness or multiple chemical sensitivities (MCS), she was **forced to change her life path dramatically.** She experienced many ill effects physically, mentally and emotionally from environmental and **chemical sensitivities.**

She left her position as a teacher then guidance counsellor of many years in the public school system to pursue her doctoral interests in psychology and environmental sensitivities due to her illness. Her doctoral dissertation on **brain allergies** and mental health issues, a rare combination not at all known or considered even to this day in 2013, became **the first work of**

its kind in the field of psychology at the University of Toronto as well as in environmental & ecological sensitivities.

In the late 90's she discovered the power of real, organic, therapeutic grade A essential oils and the art & science of **French medicinal aromatherapy.** These precious and live-food essential oils were introduced into her practices and in all of her classes as a powerful solution to many of human kinds' ills along with her energy dowsing and kinesiology techniques.

She is certified as a Registered Nutritional coach-consultant and Doctor in Natural Medicine as well as in Holistic Energy Psychology and Essential oils sciences, Egyptian dowsing and specialized Kinesiology and Body Talk. She is Director and Founder of the DeVita Wellness Institute of Living and Learning with 27 years as an eclectic psychotherapist. She is also Director – Founder of the federally approved Institute of Energy Wellness Studies of the last 7 years. Dr. DeVita is an accomplished author of five books and an international speaker. She was trained by D. Gary Young founder of Young Living Essential Oils with over 850 hours in essential oil sciences and application and certified by him in 2007 as a Raindrop technique Instructor.

Dr. DeVita is certified in Russia as a GDV Kirlian Bio-electrographic practitioner and instructor by the inventor scientist, physicist, Dr. K. Korotkov. She holds Grand master in Belvaspata. She is a graduate from the Bio-Geometry program on the **physics of quality** with both Dr. Robert Gilbert and Dr. Ibrahim Karim (founder of Bio-Geometry) and incorporates some of the simple Bio- Geometry principles in her teachings and writings.

Real Green Essentials – making women healthier© - became one of her platforms in order to promote, educate and further the mission of greening every home in **shifting consciousness! It became her Real Green Essentials© Environmental initiative.** Hon. Dr. DeVita was knighted in November 2004 as Recipient Dame of the Sovereign Order of Knights Hospitaller of St. John of Jerusalem. In 2005, she was also appointed as Deputy Member of the Canadian Delegation for the International Parliament of Safety and Peace.

She currently oversees her private practice and continues to teach in her school programs along with international speaking engagements, trainings and essential oil lectures and book appearances - presentations. She continues to maintain membership in these environmental groups:

- David Suzuki Foundation
- Environmental Defence
- Pollution Probe
- Council of Canadians
- Environmental Working Group

- Environmental Probe

- Sierra Legal Defence Club

- Canadian Association of Physicians for the Environment

- Greenpeace

*"Blinding ignorance does mislead us.
O! Wretched mortals open your eyes!"*

– Leonardo Da Vinci

*"A dream you dream alone is only a
dream. A dream you dream together is
reality."*

– John Lennon

ABOUT REAL GREEN ESSENTIALS© WORKSHOPS

Eco Green Essentials Consultant- Workshops

Our Eco Green Essentials consultants know how important it is for women, in particular, to be educated about their everyday exposures from sink to bath to brushing their teeth.

Change and better choices can be made to natural, organic products - the real green way. To help consumers make better choices in getting out of the chemical mess we're in and to stop the destruction to our planet- a definite consciousness shift and a new generation of green lifestyle experts has emerged.

Many of these experts are committed environmentalists in their own right, who love to share their insight and offer consumers a myriad of practical tips to make better, greener, healthier choices as they wade through all the products.

Our Eco Essentials consultants trained in eco healthy living and cleaning knows that their guests will be guided to eco-friendly, organic, true plant-based therapeutic grade products, experience them and have the opportunity to purchase them at a discounted price. Real Green Essentials© Workshops covers much in the consultants training:

Common toxic chemicals found in homes

Home ratings

Questionnaire for chemical symptoms

Top-Quality organic greening and health product usage

Mold remediation

Certification as a recognized Eco Green consultant

Optional Registered Identity Badge

**Contact us for certified workshops as an
Eco-Green Consultant offered by our
Canadian Federal Approved Institute:**

**www.energywellnessstudies.com
info@energywellnessstudies.com**

To Order these Therapeutic-grade oils-:
http://vita.younglivingworld.com

or contact the person that gave you this book.!

Endnotes

CHAPTER 1

Melissa Lai et al., "2005 Annual Report of the American Association of Poison Control Centers' National Poisoning Database," Clinical Toxicology, 44 (2006): 803-932, https://aapcc.s3.amazonaws.com/pdfs/annual_reports/Clin-Tox_AAPCC_2005_Annual_Report.pdf (accessed March 24, 2013).

Lang, Susan. "Water, air and soil pollution causes 40 percent of deaths worldwide, Cornell research survey finds." Cornell University, August 02, 2007. http://www.news.cornell.edu/stories/aug07/morediseases.sl.html (accessed March 24, 2013).

Environmental Protection Agency, "Learn the Issues: Air." Last modified 2013. Accessed March 24, 2013. http://www2.epa.gov/learn-issues/air.

World Health Organization, "WHO Guidelines for Indoor Air Quality: Selected Pollutants." Accessed March 24, 2013. http://www.euro.who.int/document/e94535.pdf .

L Barr et al., "Measurement of paraben concentrations in human breast tissue at serial locations across the breast from axilla to sternum," Journal of Applied Toxicology, 32, no. 3 (2012): 219-232, http://onlinelibrary.wiley.com/doi/10.1002/jat.1786/ (accessed March 24, 2013).

The Campaign for Safe Cosmetics, "Parabens." Last modified 2011. Accessed March 24, 2013. http://safecosmetics.org/article.php?id=291.

Rub a Dub Dub...Is Cancer In Your Tub?. Network News and Publications, 1999.

Dadd, Debra Lynn. *Home Safe Home*. Tarcher, 1997.

Peakin, William. "How A Clean Home Can Kill You - Hidden Toxins Galore." *The Observer*. http://observer.co.uk.

Mandal, Veronique. "Housework Makes Women Sick." *Windsor Star*, 2003.

×°Mercola,2013-http://articles.mercola.com/sites/articlesarchive/2013/05/15/toxic-chemical-exposure.aspx?e_cid=20130515RRG_DNL_art_1&utm_source=dnl&utm_medium=email&utm_content=art1&utm_campaign=20130515RRG

U.S. Geological Survey, "Reconnaissance of Contaminants in Selected Wastewater Treatment-Plant Effluent and Stormwater Runoff Entering the Columbia River, Columbia River Basin, Washington and Oregon, 2008–10." Last modified 2012. Accessed March 24, 2013. http://pubs.usgs.gov/sir/2012/5068/pdf/sir20125068.pdf.

Environmental Working Group, "Triclosan." Last modified 2013. Accessed March 24, 2013. http://www.ewg.org/skindeep/ingredient/706623/TRICLOSAN/.

Centers for Disease Control and Prevention, "National Biomonitoring Program: Triclosan." Last modified 2012. Accessed March 24, 2013. http://www.cdc.gov/biomonitoring/Triclosan_FactSheet.html.

Environmental Defence, "Environmental Defence Guide to Triclosan." Accessed March 24, 2013. http://environmentaldefence.ca/reports/environmental-defence-guide-triclosan.

Zerbe, Leah. "FDA Considers Putting Harmful Chemical in Your Mouth." *Rodale*, 2011. http://www.rodale.com/triclosan-dangers (accessed March 24, 2013).

Health Canada, "For Your Information: Antimicrobial Resistance." Last modified 2003. Accessed March 24, 2013. http://www.hc-sc.gc.ca/dhp-mps/vet/faq/amr-ram_fyi-pvi-eng.php.

Klevens RM, et al. "Invasive methicillin-resistant Staphylococcus aureus infections in the United States." *JAMA*. 298. no. 15 (2007): 1763-1771. http://www.ncbi.nlm.nih.gov/pubmed/17940231 (accessed March 24, 2013).

Alexander Tomasz, "Multiple-Antibiotic-Resistant Pathogenic Bacteria -- A Report on the Rockefeller University Workshop," *The New England Journal of Medicine*, 330 (1994): 1247-1251, http://www.nejm.org/doi/full/10.1056/NEJM199404283301725 (accessed March 24, 2013).

VL Marlatt, "Triclosan exposure alters postembryonic development in a Pacific tree frog (Pseudacris regilla) Amphibian Metamorphosis Assay (TREEMA)." *Aquatic Toxicology*, 126 (2013): 85-94, http://www.ncbi.nlm.nih.gov/pubmed/23159728 (accessed March 24, 2013).

Joseph Mercola, "The Soap You Should Never Use -- But 75 percent of Households Do," *Mercola.com* (blog), August 29, 2012, http://articles.mercola.com/sites/articles/archive/2012/08/29/triclosan-in-personal-care-products.aspx.

U.C. Davis News and Information, "Chemical widely used in antibacterial hand soaps may impair muscle function." Last modified 2012. Accessed March 24, 2013. http://news.ucdavis.edu/search/news_detail.lasso?id=10301.

CBC Marketplace, "The Dirt on Clean." Accessed March 24, 2013. http://www.cbc.ca/marketplace/webextras/triclosan/what_is_triclosan.html.

Centers for Disease Control and Prevention, "Fourth National Report on Human Exposure to Environmental Chemicals ." Last modified 2009. Accessed March 24, 2013. http://www.cdc.gov/exposurereport/pdf/FourthReport.pdf.

David Suzuki Foundation, "The difference between sodium lauryl sulfate (SLS) and sodium laureth sulfate (SLES)?." Accessed April 3, 2013. http://www.davidsuzuki.org/what-you-can-do/queen-of-green/faqs/toxics/whats-the-difference-between-sodium-lauryl-sulfate-sls-and-sodium-laureth-sulfat/.

World Health Organization: International Programme on Chemical Safety, "International Chemical Safety Card: Sodium Lauryl Sulfate." Last modified 2008. Accessed April 3, 2013. http://www.ilo.org/dyn/icsc/showcard.display?p_lang=en&p_card_id=0502.

Parsons, Sarah. "Why the U.S. Government Won't Protect Us From Toxic Chemicals In Our Food Supply." *GOOD*, February 07, 2012. http://www.

good.is/posts/why-the-u-s-government-won-t-protect-us-from-toxic-chemicals-in-our-food-supply/ (accessed April 3, 2013).

Energy Justice Network, "Dioxins & Furans: The Most Toxic Chemicals Known to Science." Last modified 2012. Accessed April 3, 2013. http://www.ejnet.org/dioxin/.

The Center for Health, Environment & Justice, "The American People's Dioxin Report." Accessed April 3, 2013. http://chej.org/wp-content/uploads/Documents/American Peoples Dioxin Report.pdf.

World Health Organization: International Agency for Research on Cancer, "Agents Classified by the IARC Monographs, Volumes 1–106." Last modified 2012. Accessed April 3, 2013. http://monographs.iarc.fr/ENG/Classification/ClassificationsAlphaOrder.pdf.

Epstein, Samuel. *Unreasonable Risk*. Environmental Toxicology, Inc., 2001.

Richard Denison, "No way to treat our kids: Formaldehyde, flame retardants and other toxics exceed safe levels in air and dust in day care centers," *Environmental Defense Fund: Chemicals and Nanomaterials*(blog), October 27, 2012, http://blogs.edf.org/nanotechnology/2012/10/25/no-way-to-treat-our-kids-formaldehyde-flame-retardants-and-other-toxics-exceed-safe-levels-in-air-and-dust-in-day-care-centers/.

Gabriel, Julie. *The Green Beauty Guide: Your Essential Resource to Organic and Natural Skin Care, Hair Care, Makeup, and Fragrances*. HCI, 2008.

Environmental Working Group, "Cleaners Database: Hall of Shame." Last modified 2013. Accessed April 3, 2013. http://www.ewg.org/cleaners/hallofshame/.

Kristof, Nicholas. "How Chemicals Affect Us." *The New York Times*, , sec. Op-Ed, May 02, 2012. http://www.nytimes.com/2012/05/03/opinion/kristof-how-chemicals-change-us.html?_r=0 (accessed March 24, 2013).

Assessing Chemical Risk: Societies Offer Expertise."*Science Magazine*, March 04, 2011. http://www.dbs.nus.edu.sg/lab/cons-lab/documents/Gibson_Sodhi_Science_2011.pdf (accessed March 24, 2013).

"New York Times' Kristof Lays Out The Case Against Endocrine Disruptors." *Enviroblog* (blog), May 03, 2012. http://www.ewg.org/enviroblog/2012/05/new-york-times-kristof-lays-out-case-against-endocrine-disruptors (accessed March 24, 2013).

Toppari, J. "Male reproductive health and environmental xenoestrogens." *Environmental Health Perspectives.* 104. no. Suppl. 4 (1995): 741-803. http://www.ncbi.nlm.nih.gov/pmc/articles/PMC1469672/ (accessed April 3, 2013).

DeVita, Sabina. *Saving Face.* The Wellness Institute of Living and Learning, 2003.

Centers for Disease Control and Prevention, "National Biomonitoring Program Factsheet: BPA." Last modified 2012. Accessed April 3, 2013. http://www.cdc.gov/biomonitoring/BisphenolA_FactSheet.html.

vom Sall, FS. "Chapel Hill bisphenol A expert panel consensus statement: integration of mechanisms, effects in animals and potential to impact human health at current levels of exposure." *Reproductive Toxicology.* 24. no. 2 (2007): 131-138. http://www.ncbi.nlm.nih.gov/pubmed/17768031 (accessed April 3, 2013).

CHAPTER 2

Valnet Jean, "Practice of Aromatherapy", English translation, Elbury Publishing Random House Group Co. 2011

Benson, Jonathan. "How to heal yourself physically and emotionally with essential oils." *Natural News*(blog), February 21, 2013. http://www.naturalnews.com/039183_essential_oils_emotional_healing_rejuvenation.html (accessed March 27, 2013).

Mason, Russ. "Exploring the Potentials of Human Olfaction." *Alternative & Complementary Therapies,* June 2005. http://online.liebertpub.com/doi/pdfplus/10.1089/act.2005.11.135 (accessed April 8, 2013).

DeVita, Sabina. *Emotional Freedom Face-Lift.* Sound Concepts, 2010.

Hirsch, Alan R. "Nostalgia: A Neuropsychiatric Understanding." *Advances in Consumer Research.* 19. (1992): 390-395. http://www.acrwebsite.org/search/view-conference-proceedings.aspx?Id=7326 (accessed April 8, 2013).

Warm, Joel. "Effects of olfactory stimulation on performance and stress in a visual sustained attention task." *J Soc Cosmet Chem.* 42. (1991): 199-210. http://journal.scconline.org/pdf/cc1991/cc042n03/p00199-p00210.pdf (accessed April 8, 2013).

Damian, Peter. *Aromatherapy: Scent and Psyche*. Healing Arts Press, 1995.

Jimbo, D. "Effects of aromatherapy on patients with Alzheimer's disease." *Psychogeriatrics*. 9. no. 4 (2009): 173-179. http://www.ncbi.nlm.nih.gov/pubmed/20377818 (accessed April 8, 2013).

Ceccarelli, Ilaria. "Effects of long-term exposure of lemon essential oil odor on behavioral, hormonal and neuronal parameters in male and female rats." *Brain Research*. 1001. no. 1-2 (2004): 178-186. http://dx.doi.org/10.1016/j.brainres.2003.10.063 (accessed April 8, 2013).

Rho, KH. "Effects of aromatherapy massage on anxiety and self-esteem in korean elderly women: a pilot study.." *International Journal of Neuroscience*. 116. no. 12 (2006): 1447-1455. http://www.ncbi.nlm.nih.gov/pubmed/17145679 (accessed April 8, 2013).

Ober, Clinton. *Earthing: The Most Important Health Discovery Ever?*. Basic Health Publications, 2010.

Essential Oil Desk Reference, Fifth Edition. Life Science Publishing, 2011

CHAPTER 3

Kavanaugh NL, Ribbeck K. Selected Antimicrobial Essential Oils Eradicate *Pseudomonas* spp. and *Staphylococcus aureus* Biofilms," *Appl Environ Microbiol*. 2012 Jun;78(11):4057-61

Essential Oil Desk Reference, Fifth Edition. Life Science Publishing, 2011.

Kalemba, D. "Antibacterial and antifungal properties of essential oils." *Current Medicinal Chemistry*. 10. no. 10 (203): 813-829. http://www.ncbi.nlm.nih.gov/pubmed/12678685 (accessed April 3, 2013).

Environmental Working Group, "Guide to Healthy Cleaning." Last modified 2013. Accessed March 27, 2013. http://www.ewg.org/guides/cleaners.

Mudarri, D. "Public health and economic impact of dampness and mold.." *Indoor Air*. 17. no. 4 (2007): 334. http://www.ncbi.nlm.nih.gov/pubmed/17542835 (accessed March 27, 2013).

Fisk, WJ. "Meta-analyses of the associations of respiratory health effects with dampness and mold in homes.." *Indoor Air*. 17. no. 4 (2007): 284-296. http://www.ncbi.nlm.nih.gov/pubmed/17661925 (accessed March 27, 2013).

Ponikau, JU. "The diagnosis and incidence of allergic fungal sinusitis.." *Mayo Clinic Proceedings*. 74. no. 9 (1999): 877-884. http://www.ncbi.nlm.nih.gov/pubmed/10488788 (accessed March 27, 2013).

Fields, Helen. "Household Molds Linked to Childhood Asthma." *NIH Research Matters* (blog), August 20, 2012. http://www.nih.gov/researchmatters/august2012/08202012molds.htm (accessed March 27, 2013).

"Brown Study Finds Link Between Depression and Household Mold." *Brown University*, August 29, 2007. http://news.brown.edu/pressreleases/2007/08/depression-and-household-mold (accessed April 8, 2013).

U.S. Environmental Protection Agency, "Should I use bleach to clean up mold?." Last modified 2010. Accessed March 27, 2013.

Oussalah, M. "Antimicrobial and Antioxidant Effects of Milk Protein-Based Film Containing Essential Oils for the Preservation of Whole Beef Muscle." *J Agric Food Chem*. 52. no. 18 (2004): 5598-5605. http://pubs.acs.org/doi/abs/10.1021/jf049389q (accessed April 8, 2013).

Oussalah, M. "Antimicrobial effects of selected plant essential oils on the growth of a Pseudomonas putida strain isolated from meat.." *Meat Science*. 73. no. 2 (2006): 236-244. http://www.ncbi.nlm.nih.gov/pubmed/22062294 (accessed April 8, 2013).

Essential Oil Desk Reference, Fifth Edition. Life Science Publishing, 2011.

Huff, Ethan A. "The best, and worst, laundry detergents with 1,4 dioxane contamination." *Natural News*, May 22, 2010. http://www.naturalnews.com/028846_laundry_detergents_dioxane.html

Agency for Toxic Substances & Disease Registry, "1,4 Dioxane." Last modified 2007. Accessed March 27, 2013. http://www.atsdr.cdc.gov/toxfaqs/tf.asp?id=954&tid=199.

Mercola, Joseph. "Are you poisoning your household with this chore?." December 21, 2011. http://articles.mercola.com/sites/articles/archive/2011/12/21/are-you-slowly-killing-your-family-with-hidden-dioxane-in-your-laundry-detergent.aspx (accessed March 27, 2013).

Silent Menace, "Air Fresheners." Last modified 2010. Accessed April 9, 2013. http://www.silentmenace.com/-Air_Fresheners_.html.

Elliott, Leslie. "Volatile Organic Compounds and Pulmonary Function in the Third National Health and Nutrition Examination Survey, 1988–

1994." *Environmental Health Perspectives.* no. 8 (2006): 1210-1214. http://www.ncbi.nlm.nih.gov/pmc/articles/PMC1551996/ (accessed April 9, 2013).

Natural Resources Defense Council, "Hidden Hazards in Air Fresheners." Last modified 2009. Accessed April 9, 2013. http://www.nrdc.org/health/home/airfresheners.asp.

Masters, Coco. "How "Fresh" is Air Freshener?." *Time*, September 24, 2007. http://www.time.com/time/health/article/0,8599,1664954,00.html (accessed April 9, 2013).

Schaller, James M.D. & Rosen Gary Ph.D., "Mold Illness, Made Simple" Hope Academic Press, Tampa Florida 2005

CHAPTER 4

Gray, Barbara. *Secrets of Energy.* Marietta, GA: Starlight Productions, 2004.

McTaggart, Lynne. *The Field.* Harper Perennial, 2008.

"Light makes the world go round." *The Intention Experiment* (blog), July 03, 2009. http://theintentionexperiment.com/light-makes-the-world-go-round.htm (accessed April 8, 2013).

Artnz, William. *What the Bleep Do We Know?.* HCI, 2007. http://www.whatthebleep.com/reality/BleepBookCh4.pdf (accessed April 8, 2013).

Young, Gary. *Aromatherapy: The Essential Beginning.* Essential Press Publishing, 1996.

Essential Oil Desk Reference, Fifth Edition. Life Science Publishing, 2011.

Ball, Philip. "Rogue theory of smell gets a boost." *Nature*(blog), December 07, 2006. http://www.nature.com/news/2006/061204/full/news061204-10.html (accessed March 28, 2013).

Takane, SY. "A structure-odour relationship study using EVA descriptors and hierarchical clustering.."*Organic Biomolecular Chemistry.* 2. no. 22 (2004): 3250-3255. http://www.ncbi.nlm.nih.gov/pubmed/15534702 (accessed March 28, 2013).

Strassman, Rick. *DMT: The Spirit Molecule: A Doctor's Revolutionary Research into the Biology of Near-Death and Mystical Experiences.* Park Street Press: 2000.

CHAPTER 5

Vey, Gary. "The Pineal Gland — The "Seat of the Soul"?."*Waking Times*, December 28, 2011. http://www.wakingtimes.com/2011/12/28/the-pineal-gland-the-seat-of-the-soul/ (accessed April 8, 2013).

Stanford Encyclopedia of Philosophy, "Descartes and the Pineal Gland." Last modified 2008. Accessed April 8, 2013. http://plato.stanford.edu/entries/pineal-gland/.

Bowen, R. "The Pineal Gland and Melatonin." Last modified 2003. Accessed April 8, 2013. http://www.vivo.colostate.edu/hbooks/pathphys/endocrine/otherendo/pineal.html.

Airaksinen, MM. "The update of 6-methoxy-1,2,3,4-tetrahydro-β -carboline and its effect on 5-hydroxytryptamine uptake and release in blood platelets." *Acta Pharmacol Toxicol.* 43. (1978): 375-380. http://www.ncbi.nlm.nih.gov/pubmed/726902 (accessed April 8, 2013).

Dale, Cyndi. *The Subtle Body: An Encyclopedia of Your Energetic Anatomy.* Sounds True, Incorporated, 2009.

Strassman, Rick. *DMT: The Spirit Molecule: A Doctor's Revolutionary Research into the Biology of Near-Death and Mystical Experiences.* Park Street Press: 2000.

Universal Healing Tao, "Darkroom Enlightenment." Accessed April 8, 2013. http://www.universal-tao.com/dark_room/index.html.

Chia, Mantak. *The Taoist Soul Body.* Destiny Books, 2007.

Choi, Anna L. "Developmental Fluoride Neurotoxicity: A Systematic Review and Meta-Analysis."*Environmental Health Perspectives.* 120. no. 10 (2007): 1362-1368.   http://www.ncbi.nlm.nih.gov/pmc/articles/PMC3491930/ (accessed April 8, 2013).

"Impact of fluoride on neurological development in children."*Harvard School of Public Health News*, July 25, 2012. http://www.hsph.harvard.edu/news/features/fluoride-childrens-health-grandjean-choi/ (accessed April 8, 2013).

Connett, Michael. "Fluoride & Intelligence: The 36 Studies."*Fluoride Action Network*, December 09, 2012. http://www.fluoridealert.org/studies/brain01/ (accessed April 8, 2013).

Connett, Michael. "The Facts About Fluoride & Human Intelligence." *Waking Times*, November 03, 2012. http://www.wakingtimes.com/2012/11/03/the-facts-about-fluoride-human-intelligence/ (accessed April 8, 2013).

Valnet, Jean. *The Practice of Aromatherapy*. Random House UK, 2004.

Highet, Juliet. *Frankincense: Oman's Gift to the World*. Prestel Publishing, 2006.

Moussaieff, A. "Incensole acetate, an incense component, elicits psychoactivity by activating TRPV3 channels in the brain." *FASEB J*. 22. no. 8 (2008): 3024-3034. http://www.ncbi.nlm.nih.gov/pubmed/18492727 (accessed April 9, 2013).

* Whitlock, R. (1999, Water fluoridation: The truth they don't want you to know. The Ecologist, 29, 39-41

CHAPTER 6

World Health Organization, "Electromagnetic fields and public health: mobile phones." Last modified 2011. Accessed March 27, 2013. http://www.who.int/mediacentre/factsheets/fs193/en/.

Khiefets, L. "Pooled analysis of recent studies on magnetic fields and childhood leukaemia." *British Journal of Cancer*. 104. no. 1 (2011): 228. http://www.ncbi.nlm.nih.gov/pubmed/20877339 (accessed March 27, 2013).

BioInitiative, "Renowned Scientists Issue Wake-up Call on EMF and RF Radiation Hazards." Last modified 2007. Accessed March 27, 2013. http://bioinitiative.org/freeaccess/press_release/docs/aug31_2007.htm.

Perry, S. "Power frequency magnetic field; depressive illness and myocardial infarction.." *Public Health*. 103. no. 3 (1989): 177-180.

Poole, C. "Depressive symptoms and headaches in relation to proximity of residence to an alternating-current transmission line right-of-way.." *American Journal of Epidemiology*. 137. no. 3 (1993): 318-330.

Wertheimer, N. "Electrical wiring configurations and childhood cancer." *American Journal of Epidemiology*. 109. no. 3 (1979): 273-284. http://aje.oxfordjournals.org/content/109/3/273.abstract (accessed March 27, 2013).

Canada Newswire, "Toronto Hospital is First to Recognize Symptoms from Wireless Radiation." Last modified 2012. Accessed April 5, 2013. http://www.newswire.ca/en/story/994377/toronto-hospital-is-first-to-recognize-symptoms-from-wireless-radiation.

Rochman, Bonnie. "Pediatricians Say Cell Phone Regulations Need Another Look." *Time*, July 20, 2012. http://healthland.time.com/2012/07/20/pediatricians-call-on-the-fcc-to-reconsider-cell-phone-radiation-standards/ (accessed April 5, 2013).

Wrenn, Eddie. "'The biggest experiment of our species': With five billion mobile users in the world, conference calls for research into potential brain cancer risks." *Daily Mail*, April 24, 2012. http://www.dailymail.co.uk/news/article-2134382/Risks-biggest-technological-experiment-history-species-Calls-research-links-using-mobile-phones-brain-cancer.html (accessed April 5, 2013).

Havas, Magda. "Non-Thermal Effects and Mechanisms of Interaction Between Electromagnetic Fields and Living Matter." *European Journal of Oncology*. Library Vol. 5. (2010): 273-300. http://www.magdahavas.com/wordpress/wp-content/uploads/2010/10/Havas-HRV-Ramazzini1.pdf (accessed April 5, 2013).

Havas, Magda. "Health Canada Admits Safety Code 6 Guideline for Microwave Radiation is Based Only On Thermal Effects." Last modified 2013. Accessed April 5, 2013. http://www.magdahavas.com/health-canada-admits-safety-code-6-guideline-for-microwave-radiation-is-based-only-on-thermal-effects/.

Kovach, Sue. "The Hidden Dangers of Cell Phone Radiation." *Life Extension*, August 2007. http://www.lef.org/magazine/mag2007/aug2007_report_cellphone_radiation_01.htm (accessed April 5, 2013).

Halgamuge, Malka. "PINEAL MELATONIN LEVEL DISRUPTION IN HUMANS DUE TO ELECTROMAGNETIC FIELDS AND ICNIRP LIMITS." *Radiation Protection Dosimetry*. (2012). http://rpd.oxfordjournals.org/content/early/2012/10/09/rpd.ncs255.abstract - (accessed April 5, 2013).

Wilson, Bary. "Evidence for an Effect of ELF Electromagnetic Fields on Human Pineal Gland Function." *Journal of Pineal Gland Research*. 9. (1990): 259-269. http://efile.mpsc.state.mi.us/efile/docs/13934/0073.pdf (accessed April 5, 2013).

Pfluger, DH. "Effects of exposure to 16.7 Hz magnetic fields on urinary 6-hydroxymelatonin sulfate excretion of Swiss railway workers." *Journal of Pineal Research*. 21. no. 2 (1996): 91-100. http://www.ncbi.nlm.nih.gov/pubmed/8912234 (accessed April 5, 2013).

CHAPTER 7

Essential Oil Desk Reference, Fifth Edition. Life Science Publishing, 2011

US EPA, http://www.epa.gov

Close, Edward, http://moldrx4u.com

CHAPTER 8

Exley, C. "Aluminium in human breast tissue.." *Journal of Inorganic Chemistry*. 101. no. 9 (2007): 1344-1346. http://www.ncbi.nlm.nih.gov/pubmed/17629949 (accessed March 29, 2013).

Mercola, Joseph. "99 percent of Breast Cancer Tissue Contained This Everyday Chemical (NOT Aluminum)." May 24, 2012. http://articles.mercola.com/sites/articles/archive/2012/05/24/parabens-on-risk-of-breast-cancer.aspx (accessed March 29, 2013).

CHAPTER 9

Main, Emily. "How to Stay Bug Free without Dangerous DEET." *Rodale*, . http://www.rodale.com/mosquito-repellants-without-deet (accessed April 9, 2013).

Abou-Donia, MB. "Co-exposure to pyridostigmine bromide, DEET, and/or permethrin causes sensorimotor deficit and alterations in brain acetylcholinesterase activity." *Pharmacol Biochem Behav*. no. 2 (2004): 253-262. http://www.ncbi.nlm.nih.gov/pubmed/14751452 (accessed April 9, 2013).

US EPA, "Permethrin Facts (RED Fact Sheet)." Accessed April 9, 2013. http://www.epa.gov/oppsrrd1/REDs/factsheets/permethrin_fs.htm.

Environmental Health, "Hazards of DEET." Last modified 2003. Accessed April 9, 2013. http://www.environmentalhealth.ca/spring03hazards.html.

Stanczyk, Nina. "Aedes aegypti Mosquitoes Exhibit Decreased Repellency by DEET following Previous Exposure." *PLOS One*. (2013). http://www.plosone.org/article/info:doi/10.1371/journal.pone.0054438 (accessed April 9, 2013).

Qualls, WA. "Field evaluation of commercial repellents against the floodwater mosquito Psorophora columbiae (Diptera: Culicidae) in St. Johns County, Florida." *Journal of Medical Entomology*. no. 6 (2011): 1247-1249. http://www.ncbi.nlm.nih.gov/pubmed/22238886 (accessed April 9, 2013).

Centers for Disease Control and Prevention, "Insect Repellent Use and Safety." Accessed April 9, 2013. http://www.cdc.gov/ncidod/dvbid/westnile/qa/insect_repellent.htm.

Gabriel, Julie. *The Green Beauty Guide: Your Essential Resource to Organic and Natural Skin Care, Hair Care, Makeup, and Fragrances*. HCI, 2008.

Mercola, Joseph. "Cinnamon Oil Better for Killing Mosquitoes Than DEET." *Mercola.com*, August 07, 2004. http://articles.mercola.com/sites/articles/archive/2004/08/07/cinnamon-oil-deet.aspx (accessed April 9, 2013).